Music Therapy in Palliative Care

of related interest

Research and Practice in Medicine
From Out of the Silence
David Aldridge
ISBN 1 85302 296 9

Music Therapy in Palliative Care
New Voices
Edited by David Aldridge
ISBN 1 85302 739 1

Spirituality, Healing and Medicine
Return to the Silence
David Aldridge
ISBN 1 85302 554 2

Music, Music Therapy and Trauma
International Perspectives
Edited by Julie P. Sutton
ISBN 1 84310 027 4

Clinical Applications of
Music Therapy in Psychiatry
Edited by Tony Wigram and Jos De Backer
Foreword by Jan Peuskens
ISBN 1 85302 733 2

Understanding Dementia
The Man with the Worried Eyes
Richard Cheston and Michael Bender
ISBN 1 85302 479 1

Healing Arts Therapies and
Person-Centred Dementia Care
Edited by Anthea Innes and Karen Hatfield
ISBN 1 84310 038 X
Bradford Dementia Group

Storymaking and Creative Groupwork
with Older People
Paula Crimmens
ISBN 1 85302 440 6

Music Therapy in Palliative Care

New Voices

Edited by David Aldridge

Jessica Kingsley Publishers
London and Philadelphia

Grateful acknowledgement is made to Pantheon Books, a Division of Random House, Inc. for permission to reprint an extract on p.25 from *The Method of Zen* by E. Herrigel, copyright © 1988 by E. Herrigel. Chapter 3 reprinted with permission from the *Journal of Music Therapy*. Originally published in the *Journal of Music Therapy, 33* (2), 1996, 74–92. All rights reserved. Extract on p.95 from *The Mozart Effect* by Don Campbell, copyright © 1997 by Don Campbell, reprinted by permission of Avon Books, Inc. Extracts on pp.105, 125 from *Doctor Faustus* by Thomas Mann, 1949, reproduced by kind permission of Secker and Warburg, Random House UK Ltd. and Alfred A. Knopf Inc., a division of Random House, Inc., New York. Extracts on p.107, 108, 114 reproduced from *On Watch – Views from the Lighthouse* by Christopher Spence, 1996, by permission of Cassell, Wellington House, 125 Strand, London WC2R 0BB. Extract on p.110 reproduced from *Dog Days, White Nights* by David Rees, 1991, by permisssion of Third House Publishing, Exeter. Extract on p.116 from *Collected Poems* by Robert Frost, 1930, reproduced with the kind permission of the estate of Robert Frost, the editor Edward Connery Lathern and Jonathan Cape Ltd., London. Grateful acknowledgement is made to Anne Harrington to reprint her poem *Jammed/Crammed/Damned* in its entirety on pp.158–159, copyright © 1997 by Anne Harrington.

First published in the United Kingdom in 1999 by
Jessica Kingsley Publishers, 116 Pentonville Road
London N1 9JB, UK
and
400 Market Street, Philadelphia, PA 19106, U S A
www.jkp.com

Copyright © Jessica Kingsley Publishers 1999
Second impression 2001
Printed digitally since 2006

Library of Congress Cataloging in Publication Data
Music therapy in palliative care : new voices / edited by David Aldridge
p.   cm.
Includes bibliographical references and index.
ISBN 1-85302-739-1 (pb : alk. paper)
1. Music therapy. 2. Palliative treatment. I. Aldridge, David.
ML3920.M89795 1998
615.8'5154--dc21
98-45893
CIP
MN

British Library Cataloguing in Publication Data
Music therapy in palliative care : new voices
1.Music therapy 2.Palliative treatment
I.Aldridge, David
615.8'5154

ISBN-13: 978 1 85302 739 0
ISBN-10: 1 85302 739 1

Printed and bound by CPI Group (UK) Ltd, Croydon, CR0 4YY

Contents

This book is dedicated to Lizzie and Bill (F.W.) Locker
for all the music they gave me as a child

Acknowledgements

The editor would like to thank the Werner Richard–Dr Carl Doerken Stiftung for their research support that made the necessary contacts and support for this and further books possible and to the Stiftung zur Förderung der Nordoff Robbins Musiktherapie for their continuing financial support for the academic work at the Institute.

Introduction

David Aldridge

Within the past decade music therapists have developed their work with people who have life-threatening illnesses and with those who are dying. This book presents some of that work from music therapists working in different approaches, in different countries. These are new voices to the music therapy literature. Although some have written journal articles, contributed book chapters and presented at conferences, they have no complete published volume to their own names. Yet. This book is an opportunity to give those voices an additional hearing. What unites their work as presented here is a high standard of practice and the fact that I know them all personally. Knowing the integrity of these clinicians, having heard their presentations at conferences, and being inspired by that blend of enthusiasm and rigour, I had the simple idea of collecting that work together so that it could be presented to a broader readership. My hope is that other practitioners, seeing their colleagues in print, will also be inspired to write. While we have traditions of case presentation and musical excellence within music therapy, and a developing practice of research, there is a neglected tradition of clinical writing. Few of us have learnt it, many of us would like to achieve it. While modern giants of the music therapy field remain for us as writing role models regarding clinical practice, my hope is that new voices will be encouraged to add themselves to this chorale.

Working together in a creative way to enhance the quality of living can help patients make sense of dying. It is important for the dying, or those with terminal illness, that approaches are used that integrate the physical, psychological, social and spiritual dimensions of their being (Aldridge 1987c, 1996; Greisinger et al. 1997; Kotarba and Hurt 1995). In addition, how we care for the sick and dying, no matter how they contracted their disease, is a matter of our own personal responsibility and a collective measure of our humanity. Hospice care has met this multi-faceted challenge and in many of the following chapters we will read how music therapy is used in such situations.

The concept of hospice contains a philosophy of palliative care that includes comfort and symptom management and is not intended to be curative. In general, the hospice approach is to maximise the available quality of life for the terminally-ill resident in the face of impending death. Part of the treatment approach is to include the family as much as possible and help them to come to terms with the process of dying. Indeed, the careful planning of hospices has meant a creative co-operation between medical directors, caring staff, patients and their families, and architects. To achieve privacy for patients and their families, while optimising medical capability, has been a singular aim for many hospice planners. As part of this designed environment, the quality of art works and the aesthetics of the sound environment makes sense too, and this has led to co-operative initiatives between artists, musicians and clinic staff. Indeed, some clinicians believe that the physical environment has an impact on the treatment process and its outcome (Gross et al. 1998). Such considerations are not new, in the ancient Persian system traditional forms of architecture were related to rhythms in music thus defining sacred spaces within the house as within the soul (Bakhtiar 1976). Recently architects and artists have also taken up the challenge to meet the health care needs of patients (Scher 1996).

The second chapter in this book is written by Trygve Aasgaard, an experienced music therapist working in paediatric oncology, who emphasises not only working with the child but with the ward situation, friends and family members in terms of a milieu. This environmental, or ecological context, has its link with the family therapy and community initiatives that began in the past decade bringing varying practitioners, friends and families together in a common endeavour (Aldridge 1987a, 1987b). There is a rapidly developing literature related to working with children with cancer (Brodsky 1989; Fagen 1982; Froehlich 1984; Marley 1984; Slivka and Magill 1986; Standley and Hanser 1995) that also focuses on specific issues like the management of paediatric pain (Loewy 1997), hospitalisation (Froehlich 1996), and special needs groups (McCauley 1996).

A feature of Trygve's work is his focus on songs, song-writing and singing. It is this focus on song-writing that continues throughout the following chapters of the book. The other emphasis that he makes is that children are more than their disease. By offering children the chance to be creative then they become something other than patients, they become expressive beings. We hear this same theme occurring in other chapters too as music therapists work with children and adults.

In Chapter 3, Clare O'Callaghan writes from her extensive experience working with song-writing in palliative care (O'Callaghan 1996a, O'Callaghan 1996b, O'Callaghan 1993). In Chapter 4 by Beth Dun and Chapter 5 by Bridgit Hogan, we read how Clare O'Callaghan's work has inspired her Australian colleagues in their clinical practice. One of the reasons for producing this book is to show how music therapists are learning from each other and are taking the work further. It is this spirit of co-operation and development that heralds a new era for the profession.

What may be surprising is that some of the music therapists are writing in their own personal voices, not in the third person. What I have tried to encourage in these authors is that it is perfectly legitimate to express themselves as they are. There is no need to detach themselves from their experiences in an attempt to make those experiences sound valid or appear scientific by adopting a particular style. Indeed, the very strength of this work is its personal authenticity. As knowledge, it is a 'knowing how' of the dedicated practitioner not the 'knowing that' of scientific certainty. Therapists, as clinicians, are strongly engaged with their clients and patients in what is a strong personal relationship. There is an intimacy in music therapy, when two souls meet, that is important for those who are suffering.

Wendy Magee's chapter, like that of Bridgit Hogan, widens the focus from cancer care to other chronic degenerative diseases in the context of neurological disability (Magee 1995b). There is an emphasis in this chapter on song-writing as a coping strategy and on the client as musician. Clients, despite their neurological challenges, are active partners in the musical endeavour, as we will see in many of the other chapters.

Susan Weber works in Germany and is originally from the United States. She trained as a psychologist as well as being a music therapist. Hers is a moving experience of what it is to work in hospice care. Like Trygve Aasgard in Chapter 2, she provides a caring environment for the patient where music is a means of comfort. Rather than the heroics of modern medicine that seek a cure, we are reminded in these pages of the equally valid healing endeavours of comfort and caring. Indeed, what we shall return to in each chapter is a reminder of an overwhelming quality that is to be found in human interaction, that of kindness. While it may be unfashionable to speak of such things, it is kindness that is a balm of great potency (Pickering 1997).

Both Nigel Hartley and Lutz Neugebauer present work in situations with patients, or clients, who are living with the challenge of the Human Immunodeficiency Virus. There is pioneering literature in this field of the work that has been developed by Colin Lee (Lee 1995, Lee 1996) and Ken Bruscia (Bruscia 1991a) and these two chapters demonstrate how other therapists have also been advancing the use of music therapy to meet this challenge.

Gudrun Aldridge's work with a breast cancer patient reminds us of the importance of a musical element, that of melody, in music therapy. Here, too, we read how important it is for us to express ourselves. What music therapy offers is a form of expression that requires no words. Sometimes we can show what we cannot say (Roy 1997) and this extends the argument that Nigel Hartley makes in his chapter, where he argues that musical improvisation defies verbal articulation. While this is true, it prevails upon us as therapists to write about therapy and about improvisation. In this book, we find that the struggle to explicate the challenge of articulating the ineffable can be realised in clinical writing. What we have to make clear is that writing about therapy, like writing about music, is not the same thing as doing therapy or making music.

The final chapter is from an Australian writer, Rob Finlayson, working with people in various settings and encouraging them to write about their experiences. He uses poetry to provide guidance, revealing what was not known before the poem was written. Here we have the element of creative surprise that occurs in performance. As in the two previous chapters, we have an artist working with others to express in an artistic form, in this case writing, what they need to express publicly. Indeed, what appears to defy articulation can be verbally expressed, given the appropriate medium. Here lies the skill of the writer-as-therapist.

I hope the reader gathers from these varying voices the dedication of the therapist to allow and encourage personal expression in others. Enabling another to communicate is at the basis of the creative arts therapies, that this communication must not be words alone, is at the heart of music therapy (Ansdell 1995; Bruscia 1991a; Bunt 1994; Lee 1995). However, whether we use words, vocal sounds or noises, we have a being in the world that is essentially articulated as form, and in the performance of this form – I should say forming – we give creation to that which is within us. When we perform music together, or articulate a poem, then the difference between 'me' and 'the other' falls away, and that is perhaps the key to much of what we do as artist-therapists. But forming alone, as an active element is not enough, there has to be a stuff of which ideas are realised. Music is sensuous. Tones have timbre and can be heard. It is in the forming of the sensuous that we find the creative act.

In a world where emotions are expressed publicly, it can all too often seem that only the loudest, coarsest expressions are appreciated. We have within these pages a reminder that what contributes to our value are those feelings which are private and subtle. So music therapy, with its potential for the quiet and the delicate, lends itself to the exposition of that which we may call sublime.

CHAPTER I

Music Therapy and the Creative Act

David Aldridge

Each individual composes the music of his own life. If he injures another he breaks the harmony, and there is discord in the melody of life.
(Khan 1979, p.65)

My friend George was diagnosed as having a chronic form of leukaemia. We were both at that time in our mid-thirties. We both had families, each having children of the same school ages, and we both were moderately successful in our careers in health care practice. All seemed rosy in the garden. We both liked to run. George, however, decided that he needed a challenge in his life and running a marathon would be just what he needed. So, to satisfy the race rules, he went for a medical check-up. Until then he felt well enough to run. Check-ups are dangerous. Something was very wrong with his blood, he discovered. Within days he was in hospital awaiting a bone-marrow transplant. Road runner to invalid in one fell swoop.

In the hospital he couldn't sleep and asked me to help him with relaxation techniques and hypnosis that he was already acquainted with through his reading, not practice. These simple techniques worked (see Aldridge 1987a, 1987b, 1987c) and when he was first released from hospital, we talked about what other techniques could be used to combat what was to be a long and tiring series of treatments. I use the word combat here as that was exactly how George saw the task before him, an uphill struggle against an unseen enemy. That was his metaphor – a battle – from which he gained strength.

Through the following months we used guided imagery to bring about progressive relaxation and to help him through the anxiety of the consultations and to motivate him through treatment. I worked closely with his haematologist and oncologist who too were interested in how we could address the many problems facing George, as it became clear that the techniques to heal his bone marrow were without success. Each treatment would bring expectations and each set of tests would end in despair. George was a believer in technology and his beloved technology was letting him down. We also went to the same church and I guess his beloved God was letting him down too.

At that time the local church was engaged in a healing ministry. Friends and family would work with the parish priest to visit the sick, to administer the sacrament of healing and to celebrate the Eucharist, in the patient's home. This was an ecumenical initiative that brought many people together within a small community. Some medical practitioners were actively supported as the parish served a local general hospital, others were sceptical but saw little threat from a well-meaning laity. Contact with the local hospice was also encouraged as the healing ministry of the church offered long-term contact before the acute stages of dying. George and his wife were pleased to have other congregation members in their home. While the future looked bleak, there was temporary relief and always the opportunity for him to talk about what was important at the time with his friends. This could be planning the future schooling of the children, the best possible diet for promoting energy, the meaning of the sacrament of the blood of Christ (to someone with leukaemia this has an urgent meaning), or what relaxation technique to use next.

One day we knew that the bone marrow changes would not work. George was dying. His oncologist didn't know what to do and I didn't know what to do. So standing awkward and helpless in George's living room one day, I had to admit to him that I was running out of ideas. Now, how do you say that as a practitioner of any persuasion? But it was true, and George was my friend, and that made it even more tragic. Why don't you sing for me, he said. At that time I had not heard of music therapy. I couldn't chicken out and ask for a music therapist. So, I sang. We sang. We were both fans of the English folk song revival and had similar record collections. From our common geographical backgrounds we enjoyed the robustness of the Watersons.[1] We could also belt out a convincing repertoire of Church hymns even though the words may not have been entirely correct and true to the original. In that moment, music brought us to another level of intimacy

---

1   The Watersons (1975) 'for pence and spicy ale'. *Topic* TSCD462 (originally 12TS265)

within a friendship that was important. If the reader has an image of boys in a choir then he or she will not be far wrong.

We had of course prayed and meditated. I was teaching meditation techniques to other groups at that time. But music was something that we could do together, the mutuality of listening and singing had an extra dimension. And it was in the use of songs that we could explore those feelings about our lives that we would not have addressed in conversation. As Englishmen there were some things that we didn't talk about openly, like tenderness and vulnerability. Indeed, we had been actively encouraged not to talk about such things, particularly at school, as people would think we were sissies. Yet, such expressions were going to be vital because George had a family that needed his tenderness and he needed theirs in return. Expressing his vulnerability, previously disguised as irritation, would be an important milestone along his own personal way towards death.

The church group coming to visit him also sang for him too. From these songs George could plan his funeral and it was through these songs that we had our deepest personal memories of him. It was in song too that I could express to George what friendship meant to me and what happens when friends don't see each other any more.

Vision in my eyes[2]

They tell me your children
are growing much older,
you have a baby that I've never seen.
Well, I have a boy, a child of my own now,
It's almost as if the past never been.

Remember those hot final days of the summer,
we sat in your garden
and watched things go by,
the children were playing, and the cats chewed our laces,
if you didn't want there was no need to try.

Building your house
the weather still held out,
morning thru evening until we were beat,

> stopping for lunch and your home, home-made beer,
> everything seemed so firm beneath our feet.
>
> You had your painting,
> and me, I had my daydreams,
> sometimes we talked for the whole morning long.
> We settled the world and all of its problems,
> laughter in our hearts, our lives were a song.
>
> And now it's ended,
> like all things they tell me,
> without our noticing we said our good-byes,
> our friendship will last without nostalgia
> but your vision will stay, here in my eyes.

In song then we had both the possibilities for creating personal intimacy, of saying what lay upon our hearts. But, as we will see in the following chapters too, there was also a social function of shared music. Family and friends could gather together and sing with him, there were the possibilities of expression already present in well-known songs that could be activated for those who were singing.

Songs took George into the future of his funeral where he would be remembered, but we could also remember him too. Undoubtedly this helped us in our grieving. But there is another important factor in that when I hear those songs today, I remember our friendship, George and his family, in all its depth and closeness. This reminiscence is also important for those who grieve and remain.

Dimensions of music

Music therapy, with its ability to offer an experience of time that is qualitatively rich and not solely chronologically determined, is a valuable intervention in palliative care. Music has soothing properties (Aldridge 1996). Yet music can also be inspiring and uplifting (see Table 1.1). In its sacred use, music has been used to transport the listener to other realms of consciousness and is used so in the final stages of dying (Schroeder Sheker 1993). Indeed, the power of music is that it has the ability to calm us, or to stir us, in so many varying dimensions (Khan 1983) and it is this potential that music therapists bring to their work in various palliative care settings,

Table 1:1: Different dimensions of music

popular: inducing motions of the body

technical: satisfying the intellect

artistic: that which has a tendency to beauty and grace

appealing: that which pierces the heart

uplifting: that in which the soul hears the harmony of the spheres

whether they are working as receptive music therapists or creative music therapists.

Different situations will make differing musical demands and we will read about these in the following chapters. Music therapy has many facets to its practice, just as music itself has many dimensions. We know from our youth that popular music will make us want to dance. Even in later years, those same movements can be recollected when a song is heard, and with those movements come emotions, perhaps long-forgotten. This has proved to be the basis of much music therapy with elderly patients.

For others, music is the sublime elixir that satisfies the intellect. Listening to the Bruckner 'Choral Motets', some of us may find the peak of an intellectual experience where the unfolding of the musical structure combined with the expectations of the pieces in their liturgical sense brings a unity of heart and mind. Similarly, with the Brahms 'German Requiem' the combination of technique, style and musical structure married to personal expression is a musical experience offering a deep intellectual satisfaction. Knowing that Brahms wrote the piece after the death of his mother, where the consolation of death is an important feature, makes such non-liturgical non-sectarian music appropriate to working with the dying. This musical appreciation has its own validity and must not necessarily be 'therapeutic', yet it is one facet that can be incorporated into a program of care that uses music.

The simplest of music can bring another facet, that of beauty and grace. A child singing her own first composed song, improvised in the moment from a deep need, brings a natural beauty to human expression. We will read in later chapters of this book how that same dimension of beauty, in a moment of grace, occurs with adults when, from the urgency of a crisis, they sing out what lies upon their souls. And it is this beautiful urgency that pierces the heart and makes music appealing to the other. When our hearts are pierced, when we are so moved by the music we make ourselves or by music that another makes, then emotions can freely flow. This release of emotion is not simply catharsis, ventilation of feeling alone, for music therapy offers a step further. Once this flow is established, music therapy offers a suitable medium in which that flow of feeling finds expressive form.

Music therapy, with the potential for bringing form out of chaos, should offer hope in situations of seeming hopelessness, and therefore a means of transcendence. This idea of transcendence, the ability to extend the self beyond the immediate context to achieve new perspectives, is seen as important in the last phases of life where dying patients are encouraged to maintain a sense of well-being in the face of imminent biological and social loss. Even in the midst of suffering it is possible to create something that is beautiful. This aesthetic expectation of self-in-relationship is positive – it is hope made manifest (Aldridge 1996). And in doing so, some are uplifted such that they hear the harmony of the spheres. This should not be a strange concept to Western culture; the music, liturgy and architecture of Christian cathedrals was so constructed with the intent of uplifting the soul of the celebrant.

Hope, meaning and a sense of purpose

Music therapy, with its emphases on personal contact and the value of the patient as a creative, productive human being, has a significant role to play in the fostering of hope and a sense of purpose in the individual. Hope involves feelings, thoughts and requires action; in other words, like music, it is dynamic and susceptible to human influence. Hope changes too: patients knowing that the hope of a long life has gone can, however, hope that they will be reconciled to their families or hope that they can tell their feelings to their friends. Discerning these subtle dimensions of hope and offering the means for their expression is a central part of palliative care. Songs have provided an important vehicle for such expression and it has been the task of song-writers throughout the ages to express the deepest of human feelings. While the use of sacred songs has reflected the spiritual dimension, it is popular songs that reflect the everyday sentiments of ever-lasting love, missing a partner, cherishing a friend and gratitude for all that has happened.

Music therapists sing such songs at the bedside or compile tapes of selected songs for family and friends.

Memories of past events can be elicited through song. Many of us have had times when past events are linked to particular songs being played at the time. Through playing such songs we can review our lives and say what is important. From this basis, we can then talk about what happened to all those dreams and plans that we had. There are probably as many songs about regret as there are about promise. Somehow, in the expression of such emotions, using the words of others, we find a common understanding that communicate what we want to say. For those of us who are inarticulate in the face of strong emotions, pre-composed songs are the vehicle for expression. For others, struggling to find what they want to say, with their own voice, composing songs or even melodies, is another important musical activity leading to self-expression. Having the skills to use both composed and improvised material is vital to the ability of a music therapist and for this purpose they are trained.

Stimulating the awareness of living, in the face of dying, is a feature of the hospice movement where being becomes more important than having. The opportunity, offered by music therapy for the patient to be made new in that moment, to assert an identity that is aesthetic in the context of another person, separate yet not abandoned; is an activity invested with that vital quality of hope. Hope, when submitted to the scrutiny of the psychologist and not conforming to an established reality, can easily be interpreted as denial. For the therapist, hope is a replacement for therapeutic nihilism enabling us to offer constructive effort and sound expectations (Menninger 1959). Sometimes hope is not for a prolonged life but for a peaceful death reconciled with self and family.

Any therapeutic task must concentrate on the restoration of hope, accommodating feelings of loss, isolation and abandonment, understanding suffering, forgiving others, accepting dependency while remaining independent and making sense of dying. Music therapy can be a powerful tool in this process of change. Change can be accommodated within the overall rubric quality of life. While the elusive life qualities inherent in creative activities – joy, release, satisfaction, simply being – are not readily susceptible to rating scales, we can hear them when they are played and feel them when they are expressed.

Music therapy appears to open up the unique possibility to take initiative in coping with disease, or to find a level at which to cope with near death. It is this opening up of the possibilities which is at the core of other existential therapies (Dreyfus 1987). Rather than the patient living in the realm of pathology alone, they are encouraged to find the realm of their own creative being, and that is in the music. Experiencing the spirit of being human and transcending the vagaries of a failing body or a fearing mind in a fragile world, is an activity that music making, like prayer and meditation, encourages.

Contact, creativity and intimacy: living as jazz

> Classical music is the expression of a fully formed culture. Jazz, however, is the creation of people under constant pressure to conform to conditions imposed on them. (Benzon 1993, p.408)

If the progress of disease is an increasing personal isolation, then the music-therapeutic relationship is an important one for maintaining interpersonal contact. A contact that is morally non-judgmental, where the ground of that contact is aesthetic. For the sick, maimed, disfigured and stigmatised (Hall 1998), the opportunity to partake in a greater beauty is important. Furthermore, the therapeutic question is not 'What am I?', a question that lies in the realm of categorisation and cognition, but 'How am I?', which is one of being.

For many patients dying with AIDS, personal relationships are deteriorating. Either friends die of the same illness, or social pressures urge an increasing isolation. Spontaneous contacts are frowned upon, and the intimacy of contact is likely to be that of the clinician rather then the friend. Music therapy offers an opportunity for intimacy within a creative relationship. The concept of atonement – literally at one with another – allows for intimacy between us, but this does not have to be at a bodily level. We can meet together at another level and music offers a real manifestation of this. When the body is failing, and will inevitably be left behind, then the soul requires another form of contact. Some authors refer to this as 'bonding' or 'connecting' in a relationship similar to friendship (Kotarba and Hurt 1995). Music offers this relational intimacy and the relationship is both non-judgmental and equal.

Tenderness is an important quality in loving relationships. So too in therapy. The simple holding of hands while a patient dies, without withdrawing, is a powerful communication of intimate contact. Although it is corporeal, hands are being held, the contact lies elsewhere. So too in the choice of music that is played. What we choose to play, whether it be from recordings or improvised music, entails an intimacy with the deepest feelings that we can share with one another. Even when recorded on tape for others who know the patient, that intimacy can be felt. How we manage such closeness should be an important part of therapeutic training and is an essential element later in clinical supervision.

It is necessary to emphasise how important it is to keep our idea of creativity broad. A patient, when asked about the values of the various arts therapies he had recently had, commented, 'I did not want to be so intensely creative (as in the art therapy), but I did enjoy the music therapy where I could sing'. If being creative is used as a metaphor for new growth, and understood solely in its material implications, then no wonder it will be rejected by some patients for whom new growth is a sign of a deterioration in health. Creativity can be used in the non-material sense, as in making music, as transcending the moment. In this transcendence, the essence of spirituality, we take a leap which is hope into a new consciousness. The actualisation of all that remains within us, even when the material element of bodily life is decaying, is a creative act. It is the actualising that is important.

Many researchers into creativity have focused upon the product that is created, that which is actualised. What some music therapists are interested in is the process of creating rather than the product itself.

The patient is encouraged to creatively form a new identity that is aesthetic, even in the face of disfigurement. When people suffer they are under pressure to conform to the conditions of life as quoted at the beginning of this section. In music therapy we offer the chance to create new conditions and that is why I would like us to consider living as 'jazz'.

Rather than the Cartesian 'cogito ergo sum' – I think therefore I am, I propose 'argo ergo sum' – I perform therefore I am (Aldridge 1996). This reminds us that our identity, even at the cellular level of the immune system, is an active system that is being improvised anew each moment to meet life's contingencies. This is not to say that nothing remains the same, we have our personality as a recurring theme. We remain recognisable. But, we must accept that everything changes. If change in the face of challenge is the biological imperative, improvising to express ourselves anew is the existential imperative. It is in the process of performance that we consider creativity: in the therapy process itself, rather than the products of that therapy.

Rather than thinking about musical performance as entertainment by a single person, or a group for others, we have a shift here in the notion of performance as being meaningful for both sets of performing participants. People play together, one will be the patient, one will be the therapist. Creativity occurs within a cultural context of therapy where there are expected roles. These roles are built upon mutuality. While there will be a tradition of music making within the culture, reflected in the talents that each participant brings; the very performance in the moment depends upon the emergence of something new as a complex interplay of communicative resources from both participants. Creativity rests within the performers, it requires no previous composer. In this sense, what is performed will be indeterminate and variable as opposed to normative and predictable. From this perspective, we can have no fixed end-points of therapy and outcomes will be varied too. What we do have is the potential for individual development and for transcendence. Even when the inevitable outcome is death.

When we consider what patients want during the process of dying, they ask to be with their friends and families, to partake in loving, caring relationships. The need is to be fully alive even in the face of an impending death. The self can be actualised even with the threat of a curtailed future. This does not mean that suffering is ignored. Indeed, self-expression is necessary in the face of adverse experiences and suffering expressed can ameliorate that suffering. The promotion of positive feelings through the forgiveness of others and reconciliation with friends is a vital creative social act. Music therapists achieve this through making music together. Some encourage their patients to make tape recordings that their families and friends can use. Personal expression finds itself within a social matrix when those tapes are listened to or played at the funeral. Healing is done at a variety of levels, not just for the individual, but within an ecology of relationships. The reader will find this sentiment of mutuality echoed throughout the following chapters. This mutuality is relevant for the therapist, they too find consolation and healing within the music activity. Music therapy is not a form of treatment in the medical sense – it is, however, a form of accompaniment.

Expressions of the body

> Thus feelings lose nothing by not being expressed. Perhaps they even gain in sincerity and intensity the less they are verbalised...there is a fundamental communication which embraces all forms of existence and which, because of its immediacy, must abandon the medium of words. (Herrigel 1988, p.97)

The dynamic of change is a process of equilibrium and self-regulation that demands spontaneity (Tauber 1994). Achieving the new becomes an intentional act, promoting sustaining activities by creating the optimal conditions – physical, psychological and spiritual – that I call an ecology and others refer to as a milieu (Tsouyopoulos 1994; see Aasgaard, Chapter 2). Expressive arts represent such a spontaneous activity. Musical improvisation demands the maintenance of a theme that must change to gain liveliness. So are our lives improvised, from the cellular to the cerebral, to maintain our identities intact. In all such processes, listening to each other is a central method for gaining information and maintaining credibility, whether it is the cell communicating with the cell, person with person, or community with community. As we will see in the following chapters, intimacy is of importance and listening to each other is the fundamental element of that intimate togetherness.

We must return once more to the central role of the body in modern society. The relationship with the self is with the body, it is here that we have the interface of internal and external. How we encounter the unfolding of our experience is reflected in our bodies. The body tells us how language works, the meta-communication as it were. The reason that music therapy is so powerful is that it emphasises the lived body as being sensed, not only as being said. So expressing ourselves as a musical identity, or as danced piece, even as a dramatic event, may stay closer to the reality of symptoms as they are expressed. Expressive culture is the projection of the body into an expressive medium, music. Manipulation of that musical medium is playful expression, and culture is dedicated to understanding how to use that medium. Form is given to feelings and cognitions. Symptoms too are bodily expressions involving feelings and cognitions, sometimes conforming to a medical interpretation, but also demanding an existential interpretation that cannot be spoken. From this perspective, we can perhaps understand that chronic diseases are problems that are being dynamically expressed upon the stage of the body and sometimes fail to be interpreted adequately in the context of treatment. We can, however, expect that what cannot be said, can be played or sung. And, when we play or sing with that expression, then we can as therapists begin to understand what is being expressed. We join with that expressive medium in the medium of its expression, and there lies the power of musical improvisation for mutual understanding of expression, an expression predicated on careful listening.

Although symptoms are the embodiment of distress, it is in the arena of their performance that we are engaged as practitioners and researchers. The means we use to understand that drama, as medical or artistic, is questioned by those persons who want to claim an identity that is other than that of the stigmatised sick. If we enter into our understanding of the dying and the chronic sick at the level of artistic performance, as musical beings, then we are no longer meeting them *a priori* as sick patients but as mutual artists in performance. How we enter into that drama as clinicians challenges our healing identities. Marcuse reminds us (in Fischer 1997) that: 'art teaches us to accept tragedy, the past and the part of reality that cannot be changed by art. Yet, even in the face of tragic reality there exists the power of aesthetic form to call fate by its name' (p.372).

Family and friends

In our treatment initiatives, and research projects, it appears prudent to include the caregivers of the patient. While this may be alien to some individual therapeutic directions, the concerns of many patients in palliative care are: knowing what will happen to their family without them, understanding that their family appreciates them and being able to say good-bye to family and friends (Greisinger *et al.* 1997). If we consider the course of life, which includes dying, as a developmental process, that process will have a personal ecology. This ecology is relationships between people. As we will see in the following chapters, relationships are fostered through music therapy. At a time when people are dying, or their bodies are failing to offer comfort, then other considerations come to the fore. When souls communicate with each other, while being dependent upon their earthly manifestations, other aspects of being become important. These aspects are subtle. They are based on kindness, hope, forgiveness, love and about being creative. In the final stages of life, when biological imperatives fail to be reconciled with existential needs, when suffering has to be resolved as well as pain relieved, then it is music that takes us beyond words.

Coda

Patients perform their lives before us. That they are individual human beings outside of the role of a patient is vital to their identity. How we come to realise their potential as enhancing, as aesthetic, is the task of the creative arts therapist. Benzon (1993) reminds us that the evolution of an expressive culture, however we project our experiences into an expressive medium, depends upon our ability to use that medium. Hence the need for the skilled practitioner, the music therapist who can orchestrate, compose, or choreograph, with the patient.

If we wish to encourage people to do something differently, we have to understand that it will be intimately connected with their identity as people and those with whom that identity is validated. Change is brought about by influencing small groups and understanding their way of being in the world. Music therapy offers the chance to do something differently. A new identity can be performed. However, patients are not left alone to find their own way, the music therapist accompanies them.

One factor we must take into account is that the serious business of living can also be fun. Optimism and a sensual pleasure in everyday activities and situations are valuable for promoting personal health. The absence of symptoms and a sense of enjoyment coupled with a zest for living appear to play a significant role in the subjective assessment of health (Wenglert and Rosén 1995). Music has a vast potential for pleasure. Music is to be played. Play can be a serious business, as any child will remind us. Perhaps for adults too we can be reminded that play is not a trivial activity, and a little bit of fun is a powerful medicine.

What I am proposing here then is an aesthetic of music therapy which reconciles the tension between music therapy as art and as purposive therapeutic practice; that is, music and therapy combined as 'music therapy'. Music therapy, with its element of play, has a purposeless purpose and while clinicians from other persuasions may find this challenging; with current material demands for outcomes research, artists will recognise this function of play in the historical debate concerning aesthetics and the purpose of art. In music therapy, the self is actualised in a harmonious environment (Fischer 1996), not simply as a social aesthetic, but as deep ecology – a deeper unity. We as performers, patient and therapist, are realised not simply as we are but also as we can be. This is reality and transcendent reality, hope made manifest. It is also ethical. We define ourselves as we wish to be united with the world, reconciled in life and promoting an integrity of experience. Such hope then is not utopian, nor simply idealistic, as it is predicated upon a real performance in the life-world.

Thomas Szasz (1998) refers to the concept of healing with words as a moral act in that it is a mutual personal activity and involved with relationship. As a focus for therapy he suggests: 'how the patient lives, how he or she might live, and how she or he ought to live. The expert's role is to engage the clients in a process of searching self-examination, with the aim of enabling them, if they so choose, to become more free and more responsible' (p.18). He goes on to remind us that the process of therapy is an open-ended dialogue where the outcome of interaction must be left in the client's hands, eventually quoting Auden (1948) who states that although we are required to help others, the power to do so is outside our control, ending: 'The final aim of every critic and teacher must be to persuade others to do without him, to realise the gifts of the spirit are never to be had at second hand' (Auden 1948, p.13). We could just as easily substitute healing with music for healing with words.

Finally, there are two important concepts taken from the Christian Bible, reflected in other doctrines and that we have already read about here. One is that of *unity*; although we are many, we are one body (Aldridge 1987c). While many of our endeavours are to encourage others to perform themselves authentically, we can sometimes discern that what is performed by our sisters and brothers has ramifications for the way in which we have our own being. The second concept is that of *accompaniment*, accompanying along the way. In ancient times when someone asked the way in the desert, it was the responsibility of the person being asked to go along part of the way with them until they were sure that the other was headed in the right direction. So too in therapy, we are asked to go along the way with those who come to us for help. In the Christian tradition we are also asked to go one extra mile than that demanded by convention. Many of us experience this in working with the dying. We realise one body and we have to go part of the way, and sometimes further than we intended.

CHAPTER 2

Music Therapy as Milieu in the Hospice and Paediatric Oncology Ward

Trygve Aasgaard

The sitting-room of the hospice day care unit is crowded with people; patients, staff, a couple of relatives, one visitor. Most people stay for a little more than an hour, some are arriving, some are leaving after a time. Today's programme is 'Country and Western'. The theme has been proposed by a patient three weeks ago. Two female patients, one 30, the other 50 years old, have been practising singing and playing with the music therapist. One is dressed in a 'Country and Western' style. A music therapy student introduces the topic. The majority of people present participate in the performing. There is much laughter and loud singing can be heard. Björn, a patient in his forties, starts telling the story about the country-singer Willy Nelson, who, he had heard, gave away most of his money and valuables because 'you can't bring any of your belongings into heaven'. We are singing about women, love, jealousy and murder. The small room vibrates with Hawaii-guitar sounds accompanying (something remotely like) broad American accents from terminally ill patients and various members of staff.

Then the 'cook-general' enters the room, ringing a bell for lunch. The themes/experiences from 'The Musical Hour' are discussed further around a large table decorated with brown, red, yellow and green leaves. Good food, in some cases individually prepared for patients, is being served. After a period of 'no programme', quietness and relaxation, the dining room is transferred into a church, a short service is held for those interested. The liturgy is characterised by simple, beautiful texts and melodies, one especially composed at the hospice by the music therapist.

Peter and Mona are both four years old. During the last two years they have spent many months in hospital. Their common diagnosis is acute lymphoblastic leukaemia (ALL). Countless hours of uncertainty, uncomfortable diagnostic procedures, treatment, side-effects and sudden re-admissions due to minor infections. Pain and anxiety, isolation and absence from normal life, but also hope, new hospital friends and good memories. Today they have finished the two-year standard treatment of ALL. At the moment the children's oncology ward is even more busy, some would say more 'chaotic' than usual. A big celebration is under way.

Then at one o'clock in the afternoon, the procession through the ward corridors starts. A nurse with the ward banner is leading the way. She is followed by the ward brass band. Doctors, nurses and teachers play wind instruments and a drum. Children wave flags and play rhythm instruments. The music therapist conducts and blows his trombone. At both ends of a large table in the Children's Playroom, the two lucky patients are seated, dressed as if it were a birthday party. Parents and grandparents wipe away tears while videoing and receiving congratulations. Members of the band sing a specially-made song, 'Hooray, you two have been clever patients!' Gifts are given to the celebrated children and for everyone, a big chocolate cake, soft drinks and coffee. Mona is climbing a chair and starts singing the sad canon: 'No one at home, nothing to drink, nothing to eat'. People join her. The canon ends: 'Take a seat on your doorstep and sing a little song'.

Hospice and hospital: two aspects of cancer care

In this text *milieu* and *environment* are used synonymously. In English the concept of 'milieu therapy' has a long tradition, not least of all in psychiatry. 'Environment' more often describes the external conditions in which a person or organism lives, but 'milieu' is also seen as the immediate environment. A hospital often contains several different milieus. What will be regarded as one milieu, is dependent on the observer's distance from – and preconceived ideas – about what is being studied. If we look at the human side of a institutional milieu, the word *communion* could be employed to describe any mutual relationships based on shared beliefs. Indeed, all these aspects of life and conditions for life can probably be embraced in the one word: culture.

Do hospice-milieu and a children's ward have anything in common at all? In a hospice the overall majority of the patients will not live for very long; in this environment people spend (a part of) their remaining days receiving palliative treatment and care, and when the time comes, they die in peace and with dignity. Contrary to the home-like hospice environment, the paediatric oncology ward is characterised by the advanced technology and bustle of a university hospital. Curative treatment takes first priority, and the majority of patients, such as children with leukaemia, will survive.

After practising as a music therapist in such different settings for more than three years, I believe there are some important similarities which enable a common exploration of the two arenas of music therapy. My question is: 'What can the role of music therapy be when it comes to creating favourable environments?'

The aim of palliative/hospice care is not only to control pain and ease suffering, but also to enhance the life that remains. Hospice patients have their own individuality of course, even though they are terminally ill. Many are not only looking back on their lives or forwards, towards an inevitable death and 'that which is beyond'. They are also enjoying any possible good moments which remain and wanting to 'seize the day' more than ever. A holistic, religious or humanistic perspective is very often the backbone of palliative/hospice care philosophy (Doyle, Hanks and Macdonald 1993). To be able to put this perspective into practice, holistic goals must be implemented, not only in the individual arrangements for each patient/family, but in the very milieu of the institution.

Being hospitalised as a child includes being exposed to a number of *stressors*. Some of the most common possible stressors are related to how the child patients experience the hospital environment, separation from parents during some acute procedures, the need to interact with strangers, their experiences and expectations concerning painful or uncomfortable procedures, and separation from peer group and siblings in routine daily events (Melamed 1992). Problems like these represent additional burdens to the suffering related directly to cancer. Music therapists in paediatric oncology settings are very often helping children individually to cope with such challenges. A modern paediatric oncology ward is also permanently struggling between providing a milieu that facilitates the most effective, life saving, but very uncomfortable medical treatment and providing conditions for the best possible good life for patients/relatives during hospitalisation. If the ultimate goals of any treatment are set with the patient's *quality of life* in mind, it might be wise to assess the realities of the environmental aspects of treatment and care, and not just consider each service or profession as an isolated entity.

Both hospices and hospital wards can easily become arenas where illness and suffering dominate. This will affect not only patients and relatives but also the staff (Alexander 1993). The professional caregiver has to engage his or her attention to ways of obtaining a good *institutional quality of life*. This demands a high degree of inter-professional collaboration.

We may ask if music therapists possess particular properties regarding the formation and maintenance of a therapeutic milieu in the hospice and in hospital. Instead of answering directly, we will approach the question by looking at various relations between music therapy and the 'environment', formulating a preliminary definition and giving a few examples of how music therapy can be directed and practised as a milieu component in the hospice and paediatric oncology wards.

The term 'music environmental therapy': old wine in a new bottle?

Music therapists work individually with patients far more often or with selected groups, rather than being concerned with providing a 'music milieu' inside or outside institutions. If we study the history of music in hospitals, we will discover that during the 10th century in Arabian hospitals musicians were engaged in soothing pain and discomfort. They seemed to provide a general beneficial musical environment, rather than working with individual patients (Kümmel 1977). The 'Tafelmusik' which has taken place in the numerous curative baths in Europe since the 17th century, is another example of milieu therapy (or diversional therapy) where music has its natural place. As the modern, professionally based music therapy has developed during this century, the focus has been on the single client, patient, family, or defined group in schools or institutions. However, some music therapy authors have been interested in exploring new and interesting 'extended' arenas for practice, such as Stige (1993) who describes cultural engagement in the local community as an example of changes in the music therapy 'space'. Can this be characterised as 'grand scale' music environmental therapy?

Within music therapeutic practices in cancer treatment and care, there has been a long tradition of a distinctive holistic implementation of artistic elements in anthroposophically oriented institutions. The standard works of music therapy in paediatric oncology (Griessmeier and Bossinger 1994) and hospice/palliative care (Munro 1984), deal primarily with the individual patient and family. As the number of hospice out-patient day wards have increased, and the music therapeutic 'presence' has become better established in child oncology, so has there been a growing interest concerning music therapeutic presence in the 'milieu' of the institutions. Music therapy groups, with various degrees of 'openness', are no longer exceptional within hospices (Aasgaard 1996a, Aasgaard 1996b; Porchet Munro 1993; Salmon 1989; Sjåsæt 1988). Some non-anthroposophical hospital cancer wards for adults (Olofsson 1995), or weekly residential programmes, for example Cancer Help Centres (Bunt 1994) also offer their patients/families participation in music/expressive arts therapy groups. But there are still very few music therapists in cancer care, who have a particular responsibility to establish and nurture a 'music environment' within the institution. There are at least two reasons for this:

(1) Music therapists, like many psychotherapists, are generally expected to work with individuals or with selected groups.

(2) Music therapy theory and training programmes have not yet been sufficiently developed when it comes to the study, practice and research on music as a means of creating therapeutically beneficial milieu/environments.

When music therapy activities enter the 'open spaces' of institutions, music has the potential to disturb various people or other activities in the environment. When music therapists are in a public room, they will be continually observed at times by members of other professions. Sometimes they have to conduct themselves according to the high expectations of others (and themselves) as inexhaustible sources of creativity and as being able to improvise, not only musically, but also 'environmentally' in all kinds of awkward situations.

There is certainly much tacit knowledge among music therapists about the environmental influences of music on institutional life. Many music therapists are probably involved in creating therapeutic environments in institutions or in 'society', but this is not reflected in music therapy literature, reports or research. The milieu of the institution seems very seldom to be the focus of interest.

A definition of music environmental therapy

Definitions of music therapy mention clients and groups far more often than the environment. Natanson (in Janicki 1993) writes about music therapy as a planned activity that aims at 're-humanising' contemporary life-styles through the many facets of musical experience. It aims to protect and restore the client's health, and to improve both social relationships and the environment.

For the sake of simplicity 'music environmental therapy' is defined here as:

A systematic process of using music to promote health in a specified environment inside or outside of institutions.

Environment in this sense is defined as the entity, which exists externally to a person or to humanity, perceived either as a whole or as that containing many distinct elements (Kim 1983, p.80). We could use the expressions *milieu* or *culture* here to replace *environment*.

In the definition of environmental music therapy, 'promoting health' has been put forward as the general aim, thus claiming that environments, and not just individuals, can be healthy or unhealthy. David Aldridge (1996) has discussed modern identity construction with reference to music therapy. His perspective is that being recognised as a 'healthy' person is for some an important feature of a modern identity. It is interesting to apply this statement on a 'macro' level when assessing institutional milieus. Both hospices and hospitals today often express some kind of health-orientation (or quality of life) as an ideal, although the patients are often critically ill or dying. In a humanistic perspective we may say that a healthy environment is one where the dominant values are among others, love, freedom and respect for the individual. A healthy environment is one that fosters self-growth and creativity, no matter what age or physical condition, and where people are mutually helping one another to experience hope, joy and beauty. To operationalise such general and optimistic concepts is far more difficult than declaring them as practical ideals. In the cancer ward and in the hospice there is often suffering and hopelessness is not easily relieved. Disease and death can be ugly, conditions for health are sometimes poor.

The levels of music therapy practice have been classified as (1) supportive (2) specific or (3) comprehensive (Maranto 1993). In relation to hospice/ hospital environmental directed music therapy, the level of practice might be considered as *supportive*, but this kind of classification has the individual patient and not the milieu in mind. The techniques are often combinations of *receptive activity* or *recreative* categories. Music can also be combined with numerous other artistic elements. Music environmental therapy can take place in corridors, halls or common rooms, in treatment rooms or out-of-doors. To regard musical environmental therapy as a school of practice in its own right is questionable, but it certainly has a focus which is unique.

Goals of music environmental therapy

The more diverse the environmental population is, and the more inconstant it is, the less specifically related to the individual the music therapeutic goals will be. Porchet-Munro (1993) raises a timely question in relation to having participants with possibly varied, and even contradictory needs at the same time: 'Whose need is it to have music, the patient's, the family's, or the caregiver's?' (p.558).

In music environmental therapy, the individual patient should not be overlooked, but the focus for interventions should be extended to encompass all present in a defined milieu. The goals will most often be made in collaboration with other staff (or even patients and their relatives). The implementation of the goals is seldom the responsibility only of the music therapist. Sometimes the music therapist acts as an inspirer or a 'starter', or simply assists other professionals. Musical elements may play a central role or a minor role. These facts might blur pure concepts of what music therapy is and thus disengage music therapists from exploring the environmental fields of action.

The versatile nature of the music environmental 'events' makes research in this field complex. The complexity is among others factors, related to problems of finding ways of understanding the role of the specific musical elements of the events being studied. To *measure effects* (even if we could agree upon what those effects would be and how to recognise them) with quantitative parameters is probably impossible. But to study the *meaning* of music therapy activities in the environment seems far more relevant. Any meanings are connected to the experiences of people, in this case patients, relatives, staff and the music therapist's own subjective knowledge.

Questions and examples of music environmental therapy

To be able to analyse or understand this complex entity, various environmental aspects should be considered. Suzie Kim (1983), a nurse theorist, uses three characteristics as frameworks for conceptualising 'environment': (1) spatial (2) temporal and (3) qualitative (p.81).

Some environmental elements are part of the immediate milieu, having a direct impact upon a person's life, while other elements are remote. As we are living our lives, this context is more or less continually changing. A music therapist may ask: 'Can music affect our perception of spatial boundaries, or how the person experiences proximity of environmental elements? Can music bring intimacy into a big institution?'

Temporal elements encompass aspects with respect to duration and form of presence, continuity or intermittent episodes, appearing randomly or regularly. Investigating a hospice/hospital milieu, we may ask questions like:

- What is the importance of weekly sing-songs for patients and staff in this institution?

- What does it mean to the population of a ward milieu to experience the 'ward band' marching through the corridors announcing 'The Big Celebration' every time a child has her/his birthday?

- How does continuous noise from technical devices and people affect the people who have to stay in hospital day and night?

- How can music contribute to the experiences of the rhythm (or pulse) of life within these institutions?[1]

The qualitative environmental aspects may be understood as physical, social and symbolic qualities (Kim 1983, p.82). As a framework for music therapy practice, this spatial, temporal and qualitative perspective seems to be valuable for comprehending contexts related to both the individual patient and to the institutional environment.

Music therapeutic strategies related to the physical environment

Assessing the overall level of sound/noise in the environment can be a useful task for a music therapist. A milieu and the individuals that comprise it, can suffer either from sensory deprivation or overload. Music and other sources

---

1   In *music environmental therapy* the concept of 'rhythm' covers far more than the distribution and accentuation of notes in time. As rhythm can be studied on a cellular scale, it can also be studied 'grand-scale' as 'school-rhythms', 'hospital-ward-rhythms', or '(daily) life-rhythms'. The relationships between the rhythms of/in our lives and health and illness need to be continually explored in music therapy research. The composer Albert Mayr (1985) made an original contribution describing 'time-health' phenomena in an anthropological and historical music context.

of sound may have both calming or stimulating effects, features that are utilised in commercial contexts. Taped background music is employed to influence people's shopping patterns or capacity for work, but it can also be heard in hospitals and we must ask ourselves to what effect. In hospice or oncology ward settings, some patients are often hypersensitive to shrill sounds. This is probably one reason for the popularity of the lyre[2] that is used at the bedside or in small rooms. Listening to live music compared to taped music is often more effective in reducing adult cancer patients' symptoms of tension-anxiety and to increase patients' vigour (Bailey 1983). Choir chimes are often heard in the corridors of the Lovisenberg Hospice. These instruments seem to be beneficial in creating a pleasant ward atmosphere. But it is wrong to believe there is one type of music or one type of instrument that is universally preferred by terminally ill patients. Jazz-rock or spirited children's songs have also been successfully performed at the bedside, at the request of patients whom one might think wanted peace and quiet, or only discreet music.

At the Lovisenberg Hospice, for example, there was a day care unit for more than two years before the inpatient unit was opened one floor up. The staff was slightly apprehensive as to the proximity of the two units. The day care musical activities were quite often rather noisy, with playing, singing, dancing and laughing. As it turned out, this was not a problem. The majority of patients and relatives upstairs said they were comfortable with these environmental sounds.

Examples of music therapy strategies related to the social environment

The main reason for considering social environment an important factor for human health is that a successful and satisfying social life is partly responsible for health, and the quality of this social life is determined by elements of the social environment and a person's handling of social environmental forces (Kim 1983, p.89).

The making of a socially stimulating but secure environment, is a challenge for institutions where patients and families are experiencing an extremely insecure and unpredictable time of life, as is often the case in hospices and paediatric oncology wards. Music therapy sessions can be

2   The lyre is a hand-held string instrument.

meeting-points for social interaction. Some events are carefully prepared and published, but the music therapist can also create more improvised 'happenings' where those interested may participate.

'Moon River'

One afternoon at the hospice, a patient (a female pastor who is 40 years old), a music therapy student and the music therapist decide to sing and play. The patient plays the flute accompanied by a 'music-minus-one' tape. They play 'Moon River' just for fun. The sounds from the music therapy room are probably reaching 'The Smokers' Room' nearby where some patients have been sitting after lunch. A patient knocks at the door. She wants to sing too. As time passes, more and more people are finding out what is going on. The singers try to improvise second and third voices; they record and listen, trying to improve the performance, then record again and again. The tiny room is hot, smelly and crowded. Its a very grey day outside. No one seems to get tired, the singing gets louder and louder. The music therapist thinks: 'What can more be sociable than singing together?'

Many children with cancer experience loneliness and isolation, their brothers and sisters often feel they are no longer the family's centre of attention (von Plessen 1995). The siblings often have to stay in hospital too for short or long periods, because their parents must be there. In this setting, they are peripheral compared to their sick sister or brother who is being treated. Parents suffer as well. The paediatric oncology ward can be seen as a closed society, with many people stuck in a state of loneliness, anxiety or insecurity. Many young cancer patients also suffer discomfort or fatigue and establishing new social contacts is difficult for them. Some are temporarily unable to initiate social interactions. We then have to ask: 'Is it more fun to have fun together? Can music therapy bring about a more varied affective institutional milieu?' At the hospice day unit, there have been comments from visitors and relatives who find it strange or even improper for there to be so much laughter and joking in the common room.

A new song

The paediatric department at 'Rikshospitalet' is an eight-storeyed building. As usual on Tuesday mornings, the entrance hall is going to be the place for a meeting of three quarters of an hour with singing, improvising, a mini-concert, and drama. The music therapist is greeted by a mother with two children as they arrive: her daughter has come to see the doctor and give some blood specimens. She is an old friend, apparently now cured from a form of leukaemia. The little brother is 'just accompanying'. He stays with the music therapist who asks him to be his assistant today and after a short preparatory rehearsal, they head for the hospital school at the top of the building. A music therapy student follows, playing a guitar, the boy shakes a tambourine and the music therapist blows a treble-recorder. They wear medieval style hats as they enter the school. A nine-year-old girl who is bedridden with an inoperable abdominal tumour, hands the music therapist a sheet of paper. She has written another song at school. This time the text is about what she expects from the forthcoming music session in 20 minutes' time. The final words of the text are: 'We'll sing and dance, sing and dance'. 'Is it possible for the music therapist to compose a melody to the text immediately?' she asks. Her mother will come and listen.

More and more children join 'the musicians' as they walk through the surgical and leukaemia wards and then downstairs. A couple of mothers are carrying their children, a well-known song rings through the corridors. A pre-school teacher gives a message about a little boy wanting to be a drum-soloist, and another patient who doesn't dare be with 'all those people'. The music therapist is asked if he can see this boy afterwards.

A concert

Thirty people are gathered in a circle round a grand piano; patients, siblings, parents, two teachers, a nurse and a new doctor. During the following minutes, the people who are present learn each other's names, as they sing, and clap hands, performing musically and dramatically together. One father is looking rather uneasy, perhaps he perceives the environment as 'childish'? He is given a large conga and seemingly relaxes as he plays with his little boy-patient's admiring eyes on him. Half of the children are 'tied' to an infusion pump. It is far too crowded to move very much for anyone, but the majority can swing their hips a little when a four-year-old girl leads the singing of a rock-like tune. One pump starts signalling something is wrong and the music therapist tries to change the rock and roll rhythm to fit the beep-beep of the pump until a nurse manages to silence the noise-maker. Some of the children look really tired, not even a smile, and with no active participation in what is going on. The music therapist plays a short recorder solo by the renaissance composer Van Eyck. He asks the audience to close their eyes and fantasise they are in Flanders, a most beautiful city and it is a sunny day early in the morning...Nearly two minutes of silence.

Last week the medical superintendent, a very good classical pianist, held a mini-concert. Next week there will be a short jazz performance by a couple of music therapy students.

Many people pass the music-makers on their way to or from the numerous laboratories, offices or wards within the paediatric department. Some stop and listen, some participate for a minute or two. The little music-therapist-assistant boy meets his mother and sister again: 'He played so well on the kettle-drum...', I say.

Music environmental events like those described here often bring about much discussion between patients and parents. After the sessions in the hall of the paediatric section, some of the participants stay on, playing an instrument or telling the music therapist something. Parent's commentaries afterwards are frequently about 'forgetting' hospital for a time. 'Is music therapy a provider of short "time out" from an otherwise rather miserable life-situation?' I ask myself.

Examples of music therapy strategies related to the symbolic environment

A symbolic environment is composed of *shared ideas on various levels*; cultural values, scientific knowledge, social norms and role expectations. An individual's ideas, attitudes, feelings and knowledge belong to him or her as inherent parts of the personality as a social object. By contrast, 'shared ideas' are seen as representing the symbolic environment. In a strict sense, 'shared ideas' belong to no one and to everyone. The concept of a symbolic environment has meaning for human life to the extent that our behaviour and human happenings are modified and patterned by such environments (Kim 1983, p.92).

We believe there have to be *authorities* in a hospital, but this should be positive with free-flowing communication between the various groups of people working or living there. Musical activities can create new relations between the participants in a milieu. To see the *authorities* become absorbed in some artistic or musical activity, helps to humanise the impression that patients and relatives have of those in power at the hospital. When patients and parents make music together with staff, it is likely that the spirit of community is strengthened within the institution.

Patients watching the Paediatric Chamber Choir, consisting mainly of doctors (male voices) and nurses, often seem to have fun observing staff in new roles. One patient said: 'My doctors face turns quite red when he is singing'.

Many new patients at the hospice day unit are afraid of being looked upon as merely 'a (soon to be) terminal patient'. It is the duty of all the staff to be realistic and at the same time to encourage patients to expose and develop their healthy sides. At the Lovisenberg Hospice, patients can actually follow courses or develop new skills in various subjects, such as tai-chi, learning to play an instrument, to paint on glass or dance the tango.

A highly-skilled teacher is a patient at the hospice day unit. She is always full of ideas and although she has her 'up and downs', she is also interested in other hospice patients and able to share her knowledge and experiences with them and the staff members. One morning, some weeks after having started the preparations together with the music therapist, she gives a 'multi-media performance' on the theme *Death in Venice,* describing Thomas Mann's short story, showing parts of Visconti's film, playing CD extracts from Mahler's Fifth Symphony and leading an interesting discussion. She is afterwards praised as the great lecturer she still is.

Children creating their own songs are often acknowledged as good authors or composers when the songs are performed 'in public' in the paediatric ward. Tom is eight years old and during one of his very long hospital visits half a year ago due to Acute Myelogenic Leukaemia (AML), he created a nonsense verse, which very soon became a popular song. His family was immensely proud of him when the short rhyme appeared on a national radio programme. Today he has an appointment for a routine control. He enters the entrance hall in the middle of a music session with lots of people present. Tom is walking steadily towards the grand piano and places himself in front. When the music therapist discovers the boy, he soon announces the singing of Tom's excellent 'Crazy Animal Song'. The song is performed. Big applause! Tom makes a low bow and then walks smiling to the laboratory.

Very sick patients, in hospices or on children's oncology wards, must not be identified with their diagnosis. Cancer might dominate, but the disease by no means tells us everything about the patient. Institutions must continually keep this in mind when treatment programmes are planned. In the end it is a question about which values shall dominate treatment and care. Music therapy never takes place in a vacuum, in such settings the various professions are really inter-dependent. There are no antagonisms between an individually directed music therapy and one directed mainly towards the environment. The best possible music therapy in hospices and in hospital is probably a combination of the two perspectives.

CHAPTER 3

Lyrical Themes in Songs Written by Palliative Care Patients

Clare C. O'Callaghan

In the eighteen years since the landmark article 'Music therapy in palliative care' was written by Munro and Mount (Munro and Mount 1978), numerous music therapists have commenced programs in palliative care inpatient and homecare settings throughout the world. Countries with music therapists working in palliative care include Canada, the United States, Australia, Sweden, Germany and England (Lee 1995; Martin 1989). The analysis of music therapy methods in palliative care is needed so that therapists develop skills most likely to benefit patients. Song writing has been discussed as a useful method in this context (Lane 1992; Magill Levreault 1993; O'Callaghan 1990; Salmon 1993; Slivka and Magill 1986), but detailed descriptions of the procedures used by music therapists to assist palliative care patients write songs are scant (O'Callaghan 1990). This chapter presents a song writing paradigm used to facilitate 39 palliative care patients composing their own songs. The songs' lyrical contents are analysed and considered in relation to the aims of palliative care.

'Palliative care focuses on those last years or months of life when a person's death is foreseeable...' (Woodruff 1993, p.7). It aims to enable a person to live the fullest quality of life possible (Hodder and Turley 1989) by addressing their medical nursing, psychosocial and spiritual needs (Woodruff 1993). Palliative care also encompasses the psychosocial, social, and spiritual needs of the patient's family for the duration of the patient's illness and during bereavement (Woodruff 1993). In palliative care, music therapy offers non-intrusive opportunities for people to connect with and express their feelings at their own chosen pace. It fosters supportive interactions between the patients and their loved ones and enables patients to maintain some degree of physical well-being. Music therapy also offers increased opportunities to communicate with brain-impaired palliative care patients.

Music therapists use a wide variety of techniques in their endeavours to enhance the quality of life of the palliative care patients and to ease the suffering of their loved ones. Alongside song-writing these include musically supported individual counselling (Bailey 1984; Forinash 1990; Munro 1984; Whittall 1991), improvisation (Delmonte 1993; Durham 1995; Lee 1995; Magee 1995b; Salmon 1993), music to facilitate communication between the patients and their significant others (Magill Levreault 1993; Martin 1991; Munro 1984; O'Callaghan 1989b; Salmon 1993; Slivka and Magill 1986; Whittall 1991), life-review including music (Beggs 1991; Lloyd-Green 1990; O'Callaghan 1984), music-facilitated pain control and relaxation (Bailey 1986; Lane 1992; Magill Levreault 1993; Mandel 1991; Martin 1989; Munro 1984; Munro and Mount 1978; O'Callaghan 1989b), guided imagery and music (Bruscia 1991b; Erdonmez 1995; Salmon 1993; Wylie and Blom 1986), and groupwork (Salmon 1989; Short 1984).

Research involving music therapy in palliative care

Anecdotal evidence has mostly been offered to support the value of music therapy in palliative care. Exceptions include empirical studies by Bailey (1983), Curtis (1986) and Whittall (1989). Bailey (1983) found that cancer patients who listen to live performance of songs were less tense and anxious and experienced a more positive mood and more vigour than patients who listened to recordings of the same songs. She argued that the human voice, human body, and guitar music could diminish the patients' feelings of isolation and, as a consequence, change their mood for the better. In her review of 465 cancer patients who received music therapy, Bailey (1985) also found that patients generally reported a reduction in pain, improvement in mood, and improvement in communication. Studies by Curtis (1986) and Whittall (1989) indicate that music therapy may promote relaxation and pain relief in palliative care patients. A graphical analysis of 17 patients' perceived pain relief, physical comfort, relaxation, and contentment scores, after listening to recorded music, pointed to the effectiveness of music (Curtis 1986). Similarly, a decrease in heart and respiration rates amongst eight palliative care patients receiving music therapy interventions including guided imagery, deep breathing, and progressive relaxation exercises suggested that music therapy reduced these patients' levels of anxiety (Whittall 1989).

Recently, qualitative research approaches were used when attempting to evaluate the role of music therapy in palliative care. Using a phenomenological research approach, Forinash (1990) examined the role of the music therapist working with the terminally ill and concluded that it was one that: '...always focuses on serving as a companion on the patient's journey...The therapist sometimes reflects, sometimes questions, sometimes directs and sometimes listens as the patient travels on his or her journey (pp.105–163).

The study

This study used a modified grounded theory research approach to investigate the lyrical themes and categories (i.e. groups of concepts) in 64 songs written by 39 palliative care inpatients over six and a half years. Originally developed by Glaser and Strauss (1967): 'A Grounded Theory is one that is inductively derived from the study of the phenomena it represents...It is discovered, developed, and provisionally verified through systematic data collection and analysis of data pertaining to that phenomenon' (Strauss and Corbin 1990, p.23). Strauss and Corbin encourage researchers to modify the approach to suit their studies, which is what I did.

The frequency with which the themes and categories recurred in the songs were also found using a modified content analysis. When applying content analysis the researcher usually constructs categories and then searches for them in the data, tending to quantify them (Kellehear 1993). In this study however, I quantified the categories and themes that emerged from the song analyses. I did not construct my own concepts and then search for them as in traditional content analysis.

Method

Description of participants

There were 39 palliative care inpatients involved in the songwriting process. Two thirds of the participants had an advanced neurological disease (n = 26), the majority with multiple sclerosis (n = 22), and one third had cancer (n = 13). Their ages ranged from 26 to over 80. Most of the patients were aged between 45 and 65 (exact ages were not available for all of the patients). Amongst the neurological patients 9 were male and 17 were female.

Amongst the cancer patients 5 were male and 8 were female. Within the neurological patient group one third had normal cognitive functioning, one third had mild, and one third had moderate or severe cognitive impairment. All of the neurological patients except two were confined to wheelchairs. Two patients were anarthric.

All of the cancer patients wrote their songs while in bed or in a bedchair. One was severely cognitively impaired. Most of the cancer and neurological patients appeared comfortable in terms of physical symptom control.

Patients were categorised as mildly, moderately, or severely cognitively impaired on the basis of clinical observations, discussions with a neuropsychologist and, where available, neuropsychological assessment reports. Patients were classified such that:

(1) Mild cognitive impairment indicated preserved long term memory, occasional immediate and recent memory loss, especially of matters regarded as of minor importance, mild adynamia (lethargy due to a neurological deficit), mild disinhibition (e.g. beginning difficulties with impulse control; occasional preservations, occasional inappropriate remarks and beginning difficulties with abstract thinking.

(2) Moderate cognitive impairment indicated fairly intact long term memory, immediate and recent memory loss although a tendency to remember matters of significance to them (especially when prompted), adynamia, disinhibition, and difficulties in abstract thinking and problem solving abilities.

(3) Severe cognitive impairment indicated scant long term memory, if any, no immediate or recent memory, severe adynamia, severe disinhibition, and no abstract thinking or problem solving abilities.

Participants' songs

Forty-three songs were written in individual sessions and 21 by either a dyad or in group sessions. Within the individual sessions the number of songs written spanned from one in a single session to eleven written over approximately two years. Amongst the group members the number of songs written spanned from one in a single session to eight songs spanning over approximately 18 months. Three patients created their lyrics before the sessions. One anarthric, quadriplegic patient with motor neurone disease wrote the lyrics of his songs using head movements upon a microswitch attached to a specially designed computer. He communicated about the musical accompaniment via an ETRAN Board (a perspex board that relies on the patient's eye movements for communication). Another blind, quadriplegic patient memorised her lyrics until a staff member had time to write them out. The third patient wrote her lyrics out before the sessions.

Procedure for writing songs

Individual sessions were held in either the music therapy room or at the patient's bedside in either single or multi-bed wards. All of the group sessions were conducted in the wards which were comprised of three or four beds. The author's criteria for inviting patients to attend the neurological music therapy groups were:

(1) the patients experienced similar types of cognitive impairment and had similar types of cognitive functions

(2) whether the patients' personality traits (which in some patients, were likely to be affected by their brain-impairment) were comparable with the other group members

(3) whether the patients attended other therapy or received nursing attention at that time.

Session format

Within the sessions, songwriting was only one of numerous music therapy techniques offered to enhance the palliative care of patients. It tended to be offered when patients expressed deep emotion, to enable validation and ventilation of their feelings. It was also offered to encourage patients to feel a sense of achievement and pride, to enable their expression of messages to people important to them, and as a commentary about or to celebrate a significant event. Songwriting was also used to encourage cohesion and support amongst the group members (O'Callaghan 1994).

Most of the songs, especially those written by individuals took one session of up to 45 minutes to complete. The patient who was quadriplegic

Table 3.1 Songwriting paradigm

1. Offer songwriting: Songwriting was offered to the patient if it was deemed appropriate.

2. Topic: The patient was invited to choose a topic. Otherwise topics reflecting happy or sad moods, often relating to the session, were suggested.

3. Brainstorm: If the patient agreed to the songwriting the patient was encouraged to brainstorm on his/her chosen topic.

4. Ideas grouped into related themes: The ideas that emerged were grouped into related areas, usually by the therapist, in what was to become a chorus or verses.

5. Key: Major or minor keys were offered.

6. Rhythm: The rhythm tended to follow the natural rhythm of the speaking voice should the words have been spoken.

7. Mood: Preferred styles of mood were then ascertained as various musical styles were improvised.

8. Melody: The patient was invited to suggest melodies for each lyrical line. Usually he/she was given a choice of two melodic fragments for each line of the song.

9. Accompaniment, dynamics, instrumentation and voicing: Interested patients (only a few) chose the style of accompaniment, dynamics, tempo, instrumentation, and voicing.

10. Title: The patient may have then named the song.

11. Write-up, record: After the song was written out, the therapist or, if possible, the patient recorded it.

and anarthric from motor neurone disease took up to six sessions to complete each of his three songs.

Songwriting paradigm

A songwriting paradigm was developed to facilitate the patients' song writing, with variations according to their physical and/or cognitive abilities. The paradigm which is illustrated in Table 3.1 specifies eleven features of songwriting that allow patients to create songs to their maximum abilities. In eleven of the songs, the patients used the word substitution method, that is, they wrote their own lyrics to well known melodies. The individual and group songwriting sessions tended to follow the same format. In group sessions all patients were encouraged to participate and the majority decision ruled when lyrical or musical aspects were in dispute. Moderate to severely cognitively impaired patients required more structure in the songwriting approach. The author found some of the communication skills for music therapists working with brain-impaired palliative care patients helpful when assisting them to write songs (O'Callaghan 1989a). For example, they gave more responses when encouraged to think concretely rather than abstractly, and when offered brief multiple choice questions or questions that required 'yes' or 'no' answers.

Lyric analysis

Sixty-four palliative care patients' song compositions were analysed via a modified Grounded Theory approach to discover the lyrical themes within them. The intention was to systematically develop brief descriptions which encompassed all of the phenomena expressed in the lyrics. In accordance with Grounded Theory, I reflected over and over the song lyrics in an attempt to discover the recurring concepts, that is the similar lyrics expressed in the songs. Occasionally, concepts were renamed when more accurate descriptions came to mind. All of the concepts that related to a similar phenomenon were grouped together and then further condensed into categories. The categories were then further condensed into themes. The research was stopped at this point.

To generate theories within the Grounded Theory paradigm one continues this process, continuing to accumulate a wide range of purposively selected data (a process called theoretical sampling) until category development is exhausted. If I had continued my research until category

Table 3.2 Open coding example of emerging concepts and categories in the songs

A. Emergence of concepts from the lyrics of an untitled patient's song

Lyrics	Concepts
Once I could give pleasure, my music would delight	previous personal qualities
	('music' used as a metaphor);
Now it's all gone, emptiness and worthlessness	living with adversity; missing former life; feeling empty, worthless;
Times needed to adjust, to learn the new way it'll be time	needed to adjust, to move on
Discover and actualise, all lying inside of me	realise potential

B. Emergence of two categories from the concepts describing the aforementioned lyrics and other patients' lyrics

Specific Concept	Nature of Concept	Significant Concept
mother (1)**, father (1)	spouse (1) home (1) parents (1) *former life*(2)	*missing*
Category: Missing family, home and former life.		
	living with illness (MS and Cancer) (6)	*expression of adversity*
empty (1), fatigued, (1), alone (1), helpless (1) frustration (3), despair (1), *worthless* (1)	*feelings* (6)	
	lack time (1), lack strength (1), treatments/ side effects (1), gave up children (1), not being with children (1);	
of what to sing (1)	uncertainty (1), changes in relationships (1), physical constraints (1), cancer always there (1), conflict with staff (1)	

Category: Expression of the adverse experiences resulting from living with the illnesses of multiple sclerosis and cancer.

* Italics denote concepts derived from the song Lyrics in Part A.

** Numbers in brackets denote the number of songs which included the concept.

development was exhausted, I would have needed to continue analysing palliative care patients' songs until no new lyrical phenomena were found. The intention of this research was to discover the intended lyrical meanings in the songs written by the 39 palliative care patients described earlier. I did not aim to develop a theory describing the lyrics that all palliative care patients write in their songs in music therapy.

Stages of lyric analysis

The stages that guided the lyric analysis of the songs included open coding, axial coding, and alternations between open and axial coding, all which are described by Strauss and Corbin (1990). The author added two more stages: verification and finding the frequencies of the categories and themes in the songs. The following describes these stages in more detail.

OPEN CODING

This is the process of breaking down, examining, comparing, and conceptualising data (Strauss and Corbin 1990, p.61). The author developed concepts, which consisted of small phrases, to summarise the lyrical content of each song in a random manner. Initially, the songs were analysed line by line. As 'specific concepts' (e.g. empty, alone, worthless) began to recur; more abstract concepts, which were described as 'nature of concepts' (e.g. feelings), were used and the lyrics were analysed by the sentence or paragraph, or by taking the whole poem. Often patients' lyrics reflected relatively abstract concepts, rendering it possible to immediately use the nature of concept classification (for example, see how 'former life', from the song in Table 3.2 was not preceded by a specific concept denoting an aspect about her 'former life'). Also, as I progressed with the research, I was able to bypass some of the specific concepts (e.g. wife or husband) and move straight to the nature of concept classifications (e.g. spouse).

I made repeated analyses of the concepts, ensuring that they accurately represented the lyrics. The concepts that related to similar phenomena were then all grouped together into 'significant concepts'. For example, expression of adversity was a significant concept used to describe adverse 'feelings', living with multiple sclerosis and cancer, adverse 'treatments, side effects' (and the other 'nature of concepts' seen in Table 3.2). A category was then developed to encompass all the concepts grouped under the one phenomenon. For example, as Table 3.2 illustrates, the above concepts were all grouped into the category: 'Expression of the adverse experiences resulting from living with the illnesses of multiple sclerosis and cancer.'

Table 3.2 illustrates the emergence of concepts in one of the patient's songs. It also shows how the concepts derived from this song (in italics) contributed to the development of two categories. The concepts in Table 3.2 that are not in italics emerged from some of the other 63 patient songs.[1]

AXIAL CODING

This involves the process whereby data are put back together in new ways after open coding, by making connections between the categories (Strauss and Corbin 1990, p.96). Where possible, the categories that related to similar phenomena were grouped together. Single words or brief statements reflecting the content of all the related category groupings were then devised. These became the song themes. For example, the two categories of 'missing Emily, home, and former life' and 'expression of the adverse experiences resulting from living with the illnesses of multiple sclerosis and cancer' (which are presented in Table 3.2) were condensed into the more abstract lyrical theme: *'self-expression of adversity'*.

ALTERNATING BETWEEN OPEN CODING AND AXIAL
(STRAUSS AND CORBIN 1990, P.98)

Further modifications to some of the categories and themes occurred as the author continued to reflect upon how accurately the lyrics were represented by them.

VERIFICATION

A music therapy university lecturer and practitioner verified all of the concepts, categories, and themes throughout the open and axial coding stages. The verification process was deemed necessary as the patients were obviously unable to validate the author's analysis of the data and to ensure that no significant lyrics were ignored during concept analysis.

1   The complete song lyrics are listed in O'Callaghan (1994).

FREQUENCIES OF CATEGORIES AND THEMES

To analyse how frequently the themes and categories recurred in the patients' songs, a modified form of content analysis was performed. The categories and themes that emerged from the song analyses were quantified.

The frequencies of the categories in the songs were delineated by quantifying the number of songs from which each category was derived. Similarly, the frequencies of the themes in the songs were delineated by quantifying the number of songs from which each theme was derived.

Results

Themes and categories that emerged from the data

Twenty-seven categories emerged from the analysis of the 64 songs and these are shown in Table 3.3. The themes that emerged from these categories are shown in Table 3.4. It is evident that three separate categories could not be related to other categories and so yielded three themes, in other words, compliments, prayers, and imagery. The other five themes each represent at least two of the categories. The frequencies with which each category and theme occurred in the songs are also listed in these tables.

Discussion

Reflections upon the themes as they relate to palliative care

The eight themes that emerged in the lyrics of 64 songs written by 39 palliative care patients were: messages, self-reflections, compliments, memories, reflections upon significant others (including pets), self-expression of adversity, imagery, and prayers. The seven most frequently recurring categories in the lyrics were: compliments to family members, staff, other patients and friends about their personal qualities and their impact upon the patients' lives; messages of positive feelings for and experiences with people, including love, care, and that one needs people; memories of relationships with people, both living and deceased; existing in the future; expressions of the adverse experiences resulting from living with the illnesses of multiple sclerosis and cancer; descriptions of stories and nature imagery scenes; and gratitude to family members, staff and God. The following compares the lyrical themes found in this study with the aims of palliative care, which addresses the physical, psychosocial, and spiritual needs of patients with degenerative illnesses, and the well-being of their families. These comparisons suggest that song writing in music therapy can support the aims of palliative care, for both the patients and their families.

Table 3.3 List of categories and the frequency with which they recurred in the songs

Categories	Frequency
Compliments to family members, staff, other patients, and friends about their personal qualities and their impact upon the patients' lives.	32 songs, 50%
Messages of positive feelings for and experiences with people, including love, care, and that one needs people.	21 songs, 33%
Memories of relationships with people, either living or deceased.	18 songs, 28%
Existing in the future.	12 songs, 19%
Description of stories and nature imagery scenes.	11 songs, 17%
Expression of the adverse experiences resulting from living with the illnesses of multiple sclerosis and cancer.	11 songs, 17%
Gratitude to family members, staff, and God.	10 songs, 16%
Description of their relationships with their pets and with other people.	8 songs, 13%
Description of what makes them happy.	8 songs, 13%
Description of people being there for each other.	8 songs, 13%
Messages of positive wishes for people's future.	7 songs, 11%
Prayers to God.	7 songs, 11%
Reflections upon home.	7 songs, 12%
Memories of previous experiences, including those with nature and during holidays and about singers.	6 songs, 9%
Missing family, home, and former life.	5 songs, 8%
Continue to remember friends and staff including those who are deceased.	5 songs, 8%
Description of their personal and physical qualities.	5 songs, 8%
Messages of social graces.	4 songs, 6%
Description of others healthy qualities.	4 songs, 6%
Intention to realise potential or fight the cancer.	4 songs, 6%
Lullabies in which messages are given to babies.	3 songs, 5%
Messages of being with, or wish to be with, someone.	3 songs, 5%

Table 3.3 List of categories and the frequency with which they recurred in the songs (continued)

Categories	Frequency
Freedom can be experienced on beautiful days and claimed through God.	3 songs, 5%
Although sometimes uncertain about what to sing, singing increases well-being and can bring people together.	3 songs, 5%
Messages about a story of Christ.	3 songs, 5%
Messages that did/doing best one could/can in the circumstances.	2 songs, 3%
Wishes for comfort and recovery.	2 songs, 3%

Table 3.4 Song themes and frequency of songs containing the themes

Messages	in 56 songs, 87%
Self-reflections	in 42 songs, 66%
Compliments	in 32 songs, 50%
Memories	in 29 songs, 45%
Reflections upon significant others, including pets	in 20 songs, 31%
Self-expression of adversity	in 16 songs, 25%
Imagery	in 11 songs, 17%
Prayers	in 7 songs, 11%

MESSAGES

It is important that caregivers helping palliative care patients make the best use of the time remaining to them and that caregivers facilitate the communication between patients and their loved ones (Sourkes 1982). Dying patients need to feel listened to and appreciated (Seravelli 1988) and positive communication between them and their loved ones can help the latter's bereavement. In 87 per cent of the songs, patients expressed important messages, including their positive feelings for and gratitude to others.

SELF-REFLECTIONS

Sixty-six per cent of the song lyrics included the patients' reflections upon themselves and 19 per cent of the songs incorporated their reflections upon existing in the future. Although Bailey (1984) regularly found the themes of 'death' and 'peace' in cancer patients' song choices these themes were barely mentioned in this study. This could have been due to two thirds of the patients having neurological conditions. Alternatively, palliative care patients, involvement in creative activities is important for their maintenance of a sense of purpose and worth (Frampton 1986) and self-fulfilment (Connell 1989), so one may speculate that song writing encouraged some patients to think about their future living. Some of the self-reflections can also be associated with patients' personal growth. For example, in the song in Table 3.2, the composer described her need to 'Discover and actualise all lying inside of me'.

COMPLIMENTS

In half of the songs, patients complimented other people, including staff, other patients, and friends, about their personal qualities and their impact upon the patients' lives. Such lyrics would be important for patients' relatives to hear to aid in their bereavement and the patients having the opportunity to compliment other patients was possibly important for their self-esteem and sense of purpose.

MEMORIES

Forty-five per cent of the song lyrics also included the patients' memories. Various music therapists have mentioned the value of a life review process for palliative care patients (Beggs 1991) and this study revealed that song writing can promote a life-review. Butler and Lewis (1982) suggested that life review can give meaning to life and help people prepare for their death.

REFLECTIONS UPON SIGNIFICANT OTHERS, INCLUDING PETS

In 31 per cent of the songs, patients reflected upon the significant others in their lives, including pets, suggesting that many patients with end stage illnesses reflect upon their meaning for others and other people's meaning for them. Again this finding demonstrates that song writing can promote the life review process.

SELF-EXPRESSION OF ADVERSITY

In 25 per cent of the songs, patients expressed adverse experiences resulting from their illnesses. Such expressions of adversity indicate that song writing can aid in the supportive counselling of palliative care patients as it is a medium through which they can ventilate their losses and other difficulties.

IMAGERY

The imagery theme was found in 17 per cent of the songs. The expression of this theme through song writing suggests that song writing offers patients an opportunity to find some refuge from all that is going on, and that such diversion may aid in symptom control. In one song, the physical discomfort of a patient's illness was juxtaposed with the imagery of 'a forest and birds, and bees and comfort'. After playing the song to the patient the author improvised while the patient, having had her pain acknowledged, imagined being in a forest. She said that the only times she felt distracted from her pain was when she listened to this and other live music being performed in music therapy.

PRAYERS

Eleven per cent of the songs included prayers, the final theme, supporting the notion that song writing can be used by some palliative care patients for spiritual expression or reflection.

A historical perspective

The connection between death, dying, and music extends back to antiquity. People from numerous cultures including the Australian Aborigines wail upon a significant loss.

At the funerals of the Kaluli people of New Guinea melodic 'sung-weeping' based upon bird sounds is improvisationally performed by women (Feld 1990). The domestic lament is still sung in many parts of Europe and elsewhere, including Russia and Ireland, where the term 'keen' is used. Modern musical expressions of loss and grief can be found in some recent popular songs, for example 'Tears in Heaven', written by Eric Clapton 1992 (Unplugged, Reprise records) following the death of his five-year-old son, and 'The Living Years', written by Mike Rutherford 1988 (Living Years, WEA) following his father's death. Obviously song creation has assisted many people, from numerous cultures across the ages, to work through their grief during their bereavement.

Today, music therapists may use song writing in their attempts to assist palliative care patients effectively deal with the biopsychosocial issues affecting their experiences. A precedent for the use of music composition to ease the journey towards death can be found amongst the American Indians. Around the time of adolescence they each found their own death chant, via for example, a vision or a dream (Levine 1982). This was a centring technique to help them cope with adversity, enabling them to feel that they had a path to follow to the 'Great Spirit' each moment until their death (Levine 1982 pp. 25–26).

Conclusion

An analysis of the song lyrics of 64 songs written by 39 palliative care patients yielded the following themes: messages, self reflections, compliments, memories, reflections upon sight others including pets, self-expression of adversity, imagery, and prayers. A comparison of these themes with the aims of palliative care suggested that song writing in music therapy can be a worthwhile experience for some patients dealing with degenerative illnesses. The messages included in the patients' songs may also ease the suffering of their loved ones.

Saunders (Saunders 1983), who is regarded as one of the founders of the modern hospice/palliative care movement, wrote: 'The last days of living should not be seen as defeat but as life's fulfilment. It is not merely a time of negation but an opportunity for positive achievement. One of the ways we can help our patients most is to believe and expect this' (p.5).

Song writing offers palliative care patients opportunities to creatively express themes significant to their life experiences, enabling them to live out their life, and avoid existing until death.

Acknowledgements

The Masters research upon which the article is based was conducted at the University of Melbourne, Faculty of Music. The data was collected from Bethlehem Hospital, Caritas Christi Hospice and the Austin and Repatriation Medical Centre. Much gratitude to Denise Erdonmez who supervised this research and to Mary Boyle for her encouragement and comments on this paper.

A version of this chapter was first published in the *Journal of Music Therapy 33*, 2, 1996, 74–92.

CHAPTER 4

Creativity and Communication

Aspects of Music Therapy in a Children's Hospital

Beth Dun

Eight o'clock, Monday morning. I'm sitting at my desk, reflecting on the day ahead. There is a list of patients who have been referred to me. Three of them are patients I've seen before... John on the oncology ward has been re-admitted. Last time he expressed anger through instrumental work. Will his need for expression be different this time? What can I offer him? Then there is Maree on the cardiac ward. She's getting weaker each day now. What sort of imaginary world can we create together today? I pause at Mike's name. He's been on the ward in a coma for a number of weeks now. What on earth can I try today in my efforts to reach him?

With these and many more thoughts and questions I head up to the wards and the children...

I am employed by the Royal Children's Hospital as one of two part-time music therapists. We provide music therapy for children and families, and function as a resource to staff throughout the hospital. Staff such as nurses, physiotherapists, teachers, refer children for music therapy, and report that music therapy is effective in helping patients deal with many aspects of their hospitalisation.

The Royal Children's Hospital (RCH) is Australia's largest Paediatric Centre providing health care for children within the state of Victoria, nationally and from overseas. It is a core centre for research and education in paediatric health care. The Music therapy program commenced at the Hospital in 1991. The University of Melbourne initiated the program to establish a music therapy position in a paediatric hospital, and to provide a training site for music therapy students. Since 1992, the program has been funded through a variety of sources within the hospital, from external grants and the fund-raising of the Music Therapy Auxiliary.

My caseload includes children with life threatening illnesses such as cancer or brain tumours, serious heart conditions, and head injuries. The reasons why children, and their families, might be referred include anxiety, depression, pain, immobility, anger, or when the children are perceived as becoming withdrawn and isolated.

Music is important for the hospitalised child because music is:

- a familiar part of childhood
- associated with positive experiences
- easily accessible – physically, psychologically and socially
- easily controlled by people of all ages
- something which can be shared with family and friends.

Music therapy at RCH aims at enhancing the child's own unique creativity and communication capabilities through influencing children's perception of themselves within the hospital environment. Hospitalised children can become inhibited and withdrawn because of their illness and/or because the hospital environment is essentially an adult environment imposed on the child's own creative world. The instant appeal of music for most children makes it a natural medium for this creativity. Songs, instruments and musical games are familiar and a source of security in a strange setting. The novelty of new musical activities can also delight, surprise and stimulate a child.

Music therapy offers a unique avenue to express feelings that cannot be conveyed in words. It provides an opportunity to vent both positive and negative energies. It can aid relaxation and pain control. Music therapy can emphasise healthy body parts, and provide opportunities to make choices and exert control over the environment.

Hospitalisation limits the possibilities of motor activities and creative outlets for this energy are needed. Children can participate in music at any level, whether it is banging a drum or manipulating instruments and objects in a song. Even as the child's health deteriorates they can be involved in music in some way.

I take my cue from the child and family in selecting the appropriate musical experience. The process is guided in subtle as well as overt ways. Sometimes I lead with engaging songs or instrumental music. At other times I try to respectfully accompany the child beating a drum or I sing softly to comfort the child. Intervention techniques vary and evolve with the needs of each child in each session. While much of what I do is informed by established methods and techniques there is a spontaneous, creative element to the work that is based on wisdom gained from practice and intuition.

Use of songs

Songs can be used to enhance communication and creativity. The use of songs is one of the most common approaches in my work, whether it is singing, song choices or song writing. Songs consist of both verbal and musical components and therefore stimulate the cognitive, physical and emotional aspects of a child.

Song lyrics can represent verbal communication. A seven-year-old girl, who, dying from heart failure, was becoming weaker each day and a heart transplant was her only option. That was eventually ruled out, as she became too weak to survive surgery. Being very weak, she was unable to do much at all. She lay with closed eyes for most of the day. Having established earlier in her hospital admission what her favourite songs were I would sit by her bed and sing these to her. Sometimes she tried to sing along; sometimes she sang all of the song, sometimes only a word or two. Towards the end of her life she did not have the physical strength to speak but indicated her choice with a slight nod of her head and listened quietly with her eyes closed. If I stopped singing she would open her eyes, indicating that I should continue. Songs involving imagination were often used to carry her in her imagination to places she would like to go. A song called 'Katherine's Magic Horse' by June Epstein was a favourite as she could ride in her imagination the magic horse to places like 'Disneyland' and 'home'.

Songs can also provide a framework for enhanced communication, as the child may be able to express through a song issues they may have had difficulty expressing verbally. For example, an eight-year-old girl became withdrawn following surgery to remove a brain tumour. She was unable to move parts of her body and seemed scared and vulnerable. This is the song we created together:

> Why does it have to be me?
> Why can't they just let me be?
> Why do I have to do things I don't want to do?
> Why does it have to be me?

Verse 1
I hate just lying here
I'd rather be somewhere else
I hate the food
I'd rather have meals that my Mum cooks

Verse 2
I hate when the babies cry
I'd really like some peace
I hate the drip
I want it out
I just want to go home

Perceptions

Strange equipment, unfamiliar sounds and smells, technical language, strangers, bright lights and strange routines can lead to a negative perception of the hospital environment. The child may feel that they are in a helpless situation over which they have no control. Their perception of themselves in that environment may be that of a passive, sick patient to whom things happen.

I believe music can influence perceptions. Our perceptions can be influenced by music affecting us at different levels of consciousness. Most of us are aware of the influence of music: for example, when we come home uptight we put on relaxing music, or at a party we play lively music. Music can engage and encourage involvement and creativity at many different levels, regardless of the child's existing state of health.

The patients, through creating and communicating in music, no matter how sick they are, can become active participants. This can change their perceptions of themselves and as a result their physical, psychological, emotional and spiritual state may be improved.

The sick child can become aware of 'the other part' – the healthy self, that may be buried under symptoms or feelings of helplessness.

For example, a four-year-old girl immobile since an operation could not even talk or vocalise. I noticed her watching me move around the room, and so I created a song for her about what she could see, hear, feel, and think. Her perception of herself changed from an inert patient to a seeing, hearing, feeling, thinking human being.

Group music therapy

Group music experiences can transform perceptions. For example, children who are admitted to the oncology ward for the first time, after being newly diagnosed with cancer of some type, are often bewildered, confused and frightened. Their parents, coming to terms with the diagnosis, are often unable to provide the full support to their child that is needed. Attending the group music therapy session on the ward can help the child to see other children dealing with the hospital experience in a positive way and provide moral support by being with others in a similar circumstance. Parents can also enjoy participating and often need to reduce tension by having fun and laughing. By participating actively and creatively in music therapy, family members are also empowered at a time when they feel that they lack control. Our observations of group music therapy on the wards where children and their parents participate together in singing and instrumental playing include changes in response from passive observers to active participants. Parents interact with their children and seem to appreciate the child's creative engagement in the music.

Changing perceptions of the hospital ward

Engaging in music making can create new perceptions of the ward. Music modifies the environment, shaping and colouring the surrounding atmosphere.

I arrived on the ward one day, just as Kerry, a ten-year-old girl, was about to have a lumbar puncture (where they put a needle into the spine to extract fluid). It is a painful and unpleasant procedure and Kerry was crying in anticipation of the pain. The nurses gave her a choice of what support she would like in the treatment room during the procedure. She chose music and requested I start straight away before she went to the treatment room. Her tears stopped as she became engaged in the songs. We were midway through a song when they came to take her to the treatment room. We paused mid-phrase during her transportation to the room and once she was made comfortable resumed where we had left off. The song we sang asks a question of each of the participants and we involved the nurses and doctor in the song, to which they obligingly joined in:

Going on a picnic leaving right away, if it doesn't rain we'll stay all day.
What did Kerry bring?

(A gap is left for response, e.g. Kerry says 'strawberries')
Kerry brought (strawberries). Going on a picnic...etc.

The atmosphere was positive and friendly. Kerry winced and let out a cry at the times the nurse said it would hurt, but each time, after a few seconds, was looking to me for the next verse of the song and easily focused again on the singing. What was perceived to be a painful, difficult procedure was over quickly without much fuss. Instead of focusing on being the recipient of a painful procedure Kerry perceived herself as the centre of a positive and creative process. Staff appreciated the change in perception, as it helped to make their job easier.

A six-year-old boy in hospital perceived himself as a sick patient all the time. He lay weakly back on his pillow, groaning and moaning. Whenever I arrived in the ward for a music session, he would often quite suddenly, sit up, open his eyes wide, and wait expectantly for the session to begin, and was always actively involved in creating music, especially on the drums.

One day I walked into the ward and he spotted me and called excitedly 'I'm going home today!' 'That's great!' I replied. Then he looked at my guitar and musical instruments and added 'But I'm coming back in for music!'

Clive Robbins comments on the change of perception from negative to positive:

> It is important not to undervalue joy. Joy is more than fun, more than having a good time. There is something transcendent about the purity of joy, something that relates to an original realisation of one's full humanness. For a child, joy in discovering self-expression or in achieving musical creation with a therapist can be monumental. Such events bring a release from feelings of confusion, restriction, inadequacy and dependency, and from negative expectations, to generate a living, positive sense of selfhood that is fundamentally optimistic. (Robbins 1993, p.15)

Coma

My caseload includes working with patients in coma (following a motor vehicle accident, as the result of a tumour, perhaps recovery from surgery or sometimes in the terminal phase of illness, such as cancer).

Patients in coma seemingly do not respond to human contact and 'not acting' can be confused with 'not perceiving'. In this environment it is a human reaction for staff, (and even parents and visitors) to withdraw personal contact and interact with the machines. I believe staff recognise this and that is why they refer the child to music therapy, believing at some level that a different kind of contact with the child is needed.

My main aim of using music therapy with children in coma is to attempt to connect with the child within his or her seemingly unresponsive body. Using music I hope to find a link of communication, in whatever form the child can access. Sometimes I try to engage the child in any type of response that would encourage activity and awareness of themselves, others and objects. Addressing emotional and communicative needs of the child frequently appears daunting, owing to the nature of each child.

I believe it is possible to create a response within a patient and not be aware of it, as it doesn't manifest itself in observable behaviour. The response from the patient is not necessarily a measure of the success of the session. Music can have an intrinsic value of its own and does not necessarily require a response from the listener. Participation can be passive too! We accept that one of the roles a music therapist plays is to silently witness a child's music making, therefore it is also acceptable in therapy for a child to silently witness a therapist's music making.

I believe the child is aware at some level of the music. I know that during the music there are observable changes in breathing pattern and heart rate, changes in movement from ataxic to passive, or gentle, or a shift from agitation to sleep or rested state. I have experience with children who have responded vocally to music eventually.

Mike

Mike was a ten-year-old boy who had suffered a head injury and was in a coma for twelve weeks. I began seeing him for music therapy two weeks after his accident. He initially showed no signs of response to the music. As the weeks went by there were changes in heart rate and breathing patterns at significant points in the music, such as at the end of a phrase or as I deliberately took in an audible breath to begin a song. At times when he was agitated I would play soothing, gentle music and he would become calm and often go to sleep. At other times I would leave off a word at the end of a phrase and pause to give him an opportunity to respond. Initially there was no overt response, then there was an intake of breath, or some mouth movements as if he was trying to respond, but we weren't sure. Then one day I paused at the end of the phrase 'Singing ai ai yippee yippee...' (From the song 'She'll be coming round the mountain'). Mike responded with a very quiet 'ai'. I played it again and he repeated the response. The next day he sang more words in the gaps left in songs. From then on he was able to sing along to whole songs and eventually was able to initiate conversations.

By using music to link with Mike it was possible to provide a form of communication in which Mike could participate.

Music as human contact

I have also worked with children who have not recovered from coma, and have eventually died. I still hope to find a link, a form of communication, that the child can access from within their coma.

One child I worked with was in a drug-induced coma after her body collapsed from disease. She was on a life support machine. Her parents and grandmother kept a constant vigil by her bedside, waiting for her to recover. The nurses referred her to me as a gesture to the parents that they hadn't given up on life for this child. I established with the parents what her favourite songs were. She had been a lively child who enjoyed singing and dancing prior to her illness. I sang with her mother those favourite songs. There was never any response from the child, but I felt that she was aware of the music, as my previous experience with other children suggested, and so I persevered. In an environment that consisted of machines and alarms, it seemed incongruous, and yet humanising, to be singing. The child never did respond and, after many weeks, life-support was withdrawn. The parents asked for me to be present at this time. They were holding the child as life slowly left her. We sang the songs that she had known so well, and the parents and grandmother reminisced and smiled about the life of their little girl. It was a sad and difficult time for all of us, yet it was still possible to celebrate life through the unique use of music. I will never know for sure whether she was able to access the music in her coma-state, but it was an important link for her parents.

Conclusion

Working as a music therapist in a children's hospital presents many mysteries for me. It is also exciting as there is much emerging information in this field. Discovering and developing appropriate and unique communication and creativity channels through music for each individual child is challenging.

Four o'clock, Monday afternoon. Reflecting on the day, what did I learn? What can I develop? It never ceases to amaze me how it all works. What did I communicate and create? What did the children communicate and create? What about tomorrow?

CHAPTER 5

Music Therapy at the End of Life
Searching for the Rite of Passage

Bridgit Hogan

Bethlehem Hospital is owned and governed by the Sisters of the Little Company of Mary which is a worldwide Congregational Order of the Catholic Church. The hospital cares for a variety of patient populations including patients reaching the final stages of a life threatening illness such as cancer or AIDS. Patients may be admitted to the inpatient hospice or the domiciliary (that is, home based) hospice program. Medical, nursing, pastoral care, volunteer, bereavement and allied health professional services, including music therapy, are available to patients admitted to these programs. The hospital also provides similar services to patients diagnosed with progressive neurological disorders, such as Motor Neurone Disease and Multiple Sclerosis, admitted on to the Neurology Unit. However, the provision of music therapy services to these patients is currently limited. The hospital hopes to expand these services eventually.

Bethlehem Hospital has an informal relaxed atmosphere allowing staff to focus on quality of life issues for patients, their families and their friends. Emotional and spiritual needs are recognised and catered for, as well as the physical and medical needs of patients. Hospice inpatients have an anticipated life expectancy of less than three months and their average length of stay in hospital is fifteen days. They may be admitted for terminal care, symptom management or respite care which allows families and friends some time out from the relentless and often stressful job of caring for their loved ones.

Terminally ill patients may experience a range of physical symptoms such as pain, constipation, anorexia, nausea, vomiting, dyspnoea (respiratory difficulties), insomnia (sleeping difficulties), fatigue and confusion. It is, however, the complex psychosocial and spiritual needs that may be more distressing for patients to experience and families and friends to observe. These symptoms may include the fear of pain, anxiety and depression, emotional isolation, despair in the face of an advancing disease, and the need to search for existential resolution and harmony so that the patients' lives and their experiences of suffering may have some purpose and meaning.

Music therapy at Bethlehem Hospital

The Music Therapy Department consists of one full time and one part time registered music therapist as well as a music therapy assistant who maintains the audio equipment library. Music therapy services are provided to hospice inpatients five days a week and hospice domiciliary patients two days a week. Staff, volunteers, patients and their families and friends may make music therapy referrals. Indications for referring patients to music therapy may include:

- coping difficulties
- depression, withdrawal
- isolation
- difficulties expressing and/or communicating thoughts, feelings, needs and desires
- difficulties exploring spirituality and/or spiritual issues
- distressing physical symptoms (for example, complex pain problems, persistent and unexplained nausea and vomiting, anxiety and fear, terminal restlessness, insomnia, dyspnoea, disorientation and confusion, and dysphasia)
- cultural language barriers.

Once a music therapy referral has been received, patients are assessed by the music therapist within two working days. Patients usually receive music therapy at their bedsides, and families and friends may be included as well as other patients.

At Bethlehem Hospital, the ultimate aim of music therapy is to assist terminally ill patients in searching for their rite of passage by playing, or performing music. The music therapist may vary and adapt the music's elements to connect with the physical, emotional or spiritual needs of the patient that are most in need of relief. Once immediate distress has been relieved, the music therapy activity can reach out to meet other dimensions of a patient's suffering. Music therapy explores the interrelationship between these human dimensions, providing an aesthetic medium for the experience and articulation of needs and balances for these dimensions to achieve a harmonic state of physical, emotional or spiritual well-being. Ultimately, the music therapy assists terminally ill patients in finding a path of acceptance and existential resolution from which to leave their bodies, separating themselves from this world to the next.

There are a variety of music therapy techniques that can be used with terminally ill patients'. I most frequently adopt 'song choice', 'listening to music' and 'life review'.

Song choice

For many terminally ill patients the process of verbally expressing and discussing their emotions may be too difficult or too threatening. For example, if an advanced progressive disease, such as cancer, has spread to certain areas of the cerebral cortex, some terminally ill patients may experience speech impairments that prevent them from verbally communicating their emotions, thoughts, needs and desires. For other patients, it may not be typically characteristic to openly express and discuss their emotions with others. These patients may prefer to process their emotions internally or, in some cases, completely deny the need to experience and process their emotions. Finally, for some patients, the content of their emotions associated with death may be too poignant and, therefore, difficult to express verbally.

If terminally ill patients are unable to experience and/or express their feelings, thoughts, needs and desires for one reason or another, their emotional dimension may become blocked, preventing its interaction with the other human dimensions. The patients' overall human compositions may eventually become starved of emotional energy and, therefore, inhibited from achieving existential resolution, completeness, harmony and peace.

These patients may benefit from the effects of song choice as it provides them with an alternative, creative and non-threatening medium through which to experience and express their emotions. For instance, patients may choose a song because its musical mood or lyrics reflect the emotions they are experiencing or wanting to experience. A song's lyrics may also communicate to patients' loved ones what they are unable to express verbally.

Other patients may choose a song because they are comforted by the memories they associate with the song.

I find that terminally ill patients usually prefer to choose songs with which they are familiar. In an environment increasingly inhibited by a progressive illness, the opportunity to recognise music as familiar and recall a song's lyrics provides patients with a sense of achievement and greater control over their environment. Listening to a familiar song may be a stimulating experience, both physically and mentally, for these patients. It provides them with something to which they can relate and through which they can actively participate with the music therapist and others. By stimulating creative participation through familiar music, the patients' senses of self-worth and purpose are enhanced. Stimulating creative participation through familiar music provides them with an incentive and motivation to actively live while dying.

Song choice is not necessarily limited to patients. For instance, their families and friends or myself may choose songs to play or perform to them because they support or reflect their moods. In addition, the songs' lyrical connotations may assist in heightening the patients' awareness and exploration of their emotional needs.

Often resulting from song choice, patients may request to compile a tape of songs that assisted in identifying, expressing and communicating thoughts and feelings to their loved ones as well as helping them to gain insight into and reflect on the dying process. When patients experience episodes of extreme pain and fear as well as loneliness, particularly in the stillness of the night, they are often comforted by listening to the messages musically conveyed on their personalised tapes of songs that they and, possibly, their loved ones have compiled together. After the patients have died, these tapes are usually of enormous assistance to their loved ones, comforting them through their bereavement period.

Listening to music

Terminally ill patients often benefit from the opportunity just to listen to music. Music provides a structured stimulus in which patients may profoundly reflect upon and contemplate existential issues. It also offers them opportunities to experience a positive alteration to their physical, emotional and/or spiritual state of well being. These experiences may be effectively facilitated by live or recorded music. Recorded music provides patients with unconditional access to music both day and night and allows them to determine when they would like to benefit from the therapeutic effects of listening to recorded music. However, recorded music lacks the care and intimacy of another human being that is present during the live performance of music.

When I perform music to patients, the interaction of energy that occurs between the patients, the music, and myself is more personal and meaningful than when the patients listen to recorded music. In addition, performing music allows me greater flexibility to manipulate the music's elements so as to address the specific needs of patients.

Performing live music: the musical elements

Some of my clinical work has been informed by theories adopted in Guided Imagery and Music (GIM) relating to the music's inner morphology (Bonny 1978). 'Morphology is the general term for the scientific study of form and structure. The term "inner" denotes the structure within a musical selection...' (p.24).

When performing music to terminally ill patients, whether familiar or unfamiliar, I attempt to be acutely aware of, and if necessary, manipulate the music's elements (for example, pitch, rhythm and tempo, vocal and/or instrumental mode, and melody and harmony). Manipulation of the music's elements allows the music therapy to connect with the patients' human dimension(s) that may have become blocked or stuck as a result of an illness. The musical element(s) gently permeates the blockage and gives it a creative avenue through which to dissipate and eventually flow again. This allows the dimensions to reconnect and interact with the other human dimensions so as to achieve a sense of balance and wholeness.

Pitch

In her second monograph, Bonny (1978) described the influences that pitch may have on an individual. For instance, low-pitched music may facilitate positive feelings of warmth, security, and support (p.28). Music involving a wide pitch range may provide the listener with a continuing tension and release situation...opening awareness from the...uninspiring ways of life to higher aspirations and understandings (p.28). If patients are physically or emotionally distressed and seem agitated and anxious, I may use music with a relatively narrow and moderately low pitch range in order to instil a sense of security, structure and support. Alternatively, if patients are relatively free of distress and have indicated a need to process their emotions, I may use music with a wider pitch range. Providing a greater range of contrasting musical pitches, wider pitched music is often more evocative and stimulating for patients to experience. This assists in heightening the patients' awareness and exploration of their emotional, and often, spiritual dimensions.

Rhythm and tempo

Appropriate use of rhythm and tempo may also be effective in supporting and/or positively altering patients' states of well being. For example, if patients are experiencing some respiratory difficulties, breathing rapidly and seem to be restless and agitated, I may perform music where the rhythm is regular and the tempo matches their rates of breathing. Whilst maintaining a regular rhythm, I will gradually reduce the music's tempo, preferably to sixty beats or less per minute, helping to regulate the patients' breathing patterns and gently guide them to more secure, relaxed and peaceful states of well-being. Conversely, if patients have the energy and are searching for a means to more actively interact with their environment, I may perform music with a faster tempo and more diverse rhythmic patterns so as to physically and emotionally engage, excite and motivate them to participate with the music, myself and others.

Vocal and/or instrumental mode

When patients' emotional, physical and/or spiritual distress manifests in unpleasant physical symptoms, my initial aim is to create a structured and low stimulation environment over which they may regain control. Therefore, I will often perform non-vocal music as some patients experience vocal music as too stimulating. Similarly, Bonny (1978) indicated that GIM clients, 'object to vocal music. Most frequently, they claim that vocal music... interferes or interrupts the train of thoughts' (p.30). When performing or playing vocal music, terminally ill patients may attempt to process the meaning of the words or associate the sounds of my voice with a significant person in their lives, possibly triggering experiences of positive and/or negative transference. Depending on patients' needs, these experiences may be beneficial. However, when attempting to immediately relieve their physical symptoms, I tend not to sing along to the music I am performing. If I feel that patients may benefit from the energies omitted from my voice, I may hum along with the music. When conditions allow or require the need to explore, experience and express emotional, physical or spiritual dimensions, then vocal music is often more effective than instrumental music.

Melody and harmony

Appropriate use of melody and harmony may also be effective in positively altering patients' human dimensions. If I am attempting to induce a state of relaxation, I will often select music where the melody is reasonably contained, moving in stepwise motion or small intervals, and is relatively repetitive. Combined with harmonies based around the primary chords (for example, I, IV and V), the music provides a sense of security, predictability and structure (for example, 'Bach's Prelude 1'). Alternatively, if patients are requiring more stimulating music in which to explore and enhance their emotional or spiritual dimensions, I may play or perform music with more complex melodic patterns, where the melody is shared by different instruments or voices and moves in a variety of directions. I may also perform music where the harmonies are richer, sometimes unresolved and less predictable (for example, Debussy's 'Clair de Lune'). This complex combination of harmony and tempo creates a variety of colours and expectations, therefore, stimulating different emotions to experience and explore.

Whilst I give much consideration to the music's inner morphology when performing music to patients, it is not formulaic. Rather, it is a collection of musical tools from which I may select one or more when tailoring music to address the physical, emotional and/or spiritual needs of terminally ill patients.

Life-review

Life-reviews are another technique frequently incorporated into my clinical practice. As death approaches, whether consciously or unconsciously, patients often need to explore their spiritual dimensions. This may be achieved by reviewing their lives and reflecting on their achievements, failings and regrets, as well as their futures, so that they may experience a greater understanding of life's meaning.

During music therapy sessions, I will encourage patients to recall their pasts via singing, listening and playing music together and then, if necessary, discussing the associations and memories triggered by the music. Unfortunately, patients are often too ill to review their entire lives and music therapy sessions are often a series of segmented life reviews where patients recall and discuss memories from particular periods.

For many patients, music will elicit memories of significant events, people and places they have experienced. The recollection of these memories are often vivid and may be experienced through the kinaesthetic, visual and/or auditory senses:

For example:

> When you played 'I'll Take You Home Again Kathleen', my thoughts went immediately back to my Mother because that was her favourite…I could almost hear her singing it…I felt that Mum was there (pp.178–179)… Then (the music therapist) played a song that my husband and I would dance to and I just felt he was there…I felt we were going around the floor…it brought things back so vividly. (Hogan 1997, pp.215–216)

The opportunity to discuss the relevance and importance of memories and associations elicited by the music, helps patients to clarify life values. This allows patients to experience a sense of self-worth whilst giving meaning and purpose to their suffering.

Whether through song choice, listening to music or life reviews, music is capable of connecting with patients at a profound level. It shifts and balances the dimensions of their human compositions so as to creatively relieve discomfort and achieve a heightened awareness of self. The music gently guides terminally ill patients through their journey that searches for resolution, harmony and peace and prepares a path for existential transition and transformation; their rite of passage.

Case study

The following is a case study of a terminally ill gentleman, K, whom I provided music therapy to several years ago. During K's admission to Bethlehem Hospital the music therapy accompanied him on a journey in search for his rite of passage.

K was a 50-year-old male with a two-year history of high-grade astrocytoma. He was admitted three times to Bethlehem Hospital for respite care and eventually terminal care. On his final admission, K presented as overweight with left-sided weakness and occasional headaches. K's wife, L, had been caring for him at home with the support of their three daughters aged 23, 19 and 17. They were an extremely close and united family, devoted to caring for K and supporting each other.

Two years before K passed away, doctors had told him that he had a prognosis of less than six months, which K had obviously exceeded. This false time frame caused K and his family and friends enormous frustration and anxiety. During K's two-year battle with cancer, his condition constantly changed. The unpredictable nature of K's disease, his ever changing symptoms, which eventually included a personality change, confused him and his family as they experienced conflicting emotions such as loss as well as hope.

On first meeting K and L, I was overwhelmed by their sense of panic and confusion. K was in bed looking very restless and anxious and L was by his side holding his hand desperately trying to rescue him from his pain. When I introduced the music therapy and myself they were most grateful and eager for my help. I instantly felt that something was needed to calm the atmosphere. There was a need to shut out extraneous noises and dilute their sense of panic so that they could start to regain some control over their environment.

Needing to create a structured and low stimulation environment, with their agreement, I performed Bach's 'Prelude 1' then Enya's 'Watermark', as the musical elements of these pieces are conservative, structured and predictable. Initially, I performed these pieces at a faster tempo synchronising with K's rapid rate of breathing. Over time, I reduced the music's tempo and, eventually, K became calmer, less anxious and less restless. L started to appear more at ease. They seemed relieved that someone was doing something positive to them and for them, stating: 'That's lovely. That's relaxing. Thank you.'

As K and L appeared more in control of their environment, I went on to play Liszt's 'Consolation in Db Major'. This is a more stimulating and evocative piece of music as the musical elements are more complex (for example, conflicting rhythms and richer harmonies) than the previous pieces that I performed to K and L. K started to image to this piece and at its completion he talked about how it reminded him of running water and the time he and his family went on a fishing holiday. Less restless, K and L were enjoying the opportunity to reminisce of happier and more normal days.

The following day, K and L were less anxious and less restless and keen for another music therapy session. They wanted to know more about my role in the hospital. We talked about this for a while and I described other types of music I may play to patients such as hymns, old popular music, as well as songs from various stage musicals. They recognised the titles and requested that I play some of them. I performed 'I'll Be Loving You Always'. Whilst this is a very old song (written in 1925), it is popular and familiar to a lot of people. The lyrics convey an emotionally poignant and evocative message of everlasting love to which K and L were able to relate. As I performed the piece, I noticed that K and L had started to cry and held each other's hands. At the song's completion they chose not to talk about their emotions surfaced, stating: 'It just makes me sad' and 'Don't worry about us. It's just that the music brings it all to the surface.' They requested that I continue to perform more pieces. I went on to play 'When I Grow Too Old to Dream', 'Some Enchanted Evening', 'Somewhere My Love' and 'Danny Boy' (the Londonderry Air). Performed in a slow and soothing manner, K and L were able to reflect and contemplate the emotive messages such as separation, loss, love, death and peace conveyed in the lyrics of these pieces. Tearful but relaxed, K and L silently listened to the music performed maintaining eye contact with each other and frequently exchanging reassuring smiles. After I had performed 'Danny Boy', K said 'That's my favourite song. It is beautiful. I could happily die to that piece.'

During the following three or four weeks, K's health stabilised allowing him to enjoy quality time with his family. However, this was a particularly stressful time for L. Whilst grateful to share happier times with K, L felt that she was sitting on the edge of disaster knowing that at any time K could die. L would say: 'Don't think I want K to die. I just wish something would happen one way or the other. I can't stand all this uncertainty.' During this period the music therapy sessions became a refuge for L. It pleased her to see K relax and reminisce about happier times whilst allowing her to take her mind off the future's uncertainty.

The purpose of the music therapy sessions varied according to K and L's needs. Sometimes K just wanted to relax. On these occasions, I played gentle classical music and, occasionally, slow popular songs with which K and L were familiar. Performing these pieces at approximately 50 to 60 beats per minute whilst often only humming to the music, K and L frequently spent these sessions in silence, holding each others hands and usually drifting off to sleep.

Other times, they would talk about the memories they associated with the music or, asking me to sing, they would talk about the messages conveyed in the songs and the emotions evoked. These sessions were often emotionally exhausting for K and L. Therefore, I balanced them with more light-hearted sessions. Occasionally I would visit K and L without the music. This provided them with the opportunities to talk about anything they wanted. Sometimes they talked about day to day topics. Other times they talked about how they were coping with K's hospitalisation.

In the last three weeks of K's life, his physical symptoms started to worsen and he experienced a lot of physical discomfort. His speech deteriorated dramatically and he became increasingly dependent on writing down his needs, which eventually became too difficult. During this phase of K's illness he was comforted by the familiarity of music performed during previous sessions providing him with a sense of security and predictability in an ever-increasing unpredictable environment. However, sometimes the music triggered distressed responses from K reminding him of the things he wanted to express to L and his daughters but was unable to say.

I eventually suggested to K that we could compile a tape of all the songs that expressed to L and his daughters, messages and memories he was no longer able to express verbally. K was extremely keen to pursue this idea. Whilst a time consuming project, with the help of L and the girls, we were able to determine the songs K wanted on his tape. K invited all of us to contribute to his tape. This tape included 15 songs all of which conveyed messages of memories, everlasting love, peace and hope.

When K was alone at night and distressed he was often comforted by listening to his tape. Nurses would often report the effectiveness of using this tape to reduce K's pain and anxiety. I also gave L a copy of the tape. She described how listening to the tape was like reading letters K had written to her, When I want to feel close to K, I just listen to his tape.

On the morning that K died I went up to his room where L was sitting at his bedside, fearful and panic-stricken. I immediately asked her if she would like me to put on K's tape and she agreed. K had been unconscious for four days.

The first song that played was 'Memories' from the stage musical 'Cats'. The second song that played was 'Don't Cry for Me, Argentina'. Near the end of this song, L became overwhelmed with emotions and, nestling her head into K's arm, she started to cry. At this point K opened his eyes and looked at L. 'Danny Boy' started to play and after the words '...the pipes, the pipes are calling', K closed his eyes and passed away. Eventually K's daughters arrived and with L, they sat with K for a couple of hours whilst the music continued to play.

Parts of K's tape were played at his funeral. L and his three daughters all have a copy of the tape and even today, they still listen to it. L often tells me how it has helped her through her bereavement, The music has put a time perspective on K' death. It has given it a framework. With each song I am able to vividly recall what happened during his death experience which I find very comforting.

For me, this case study has always epitomised the way music therapy can support and guide terminally ill patients towards their point of departure. Connecting with the dimensions of K's human composition, the music therapy provided a creative medium for the resolution and interaction of his physical, emotional and spiritual dimensions. It helped to decrease his physical discomfort and gave him a voice through which he could express and communicate with his family. The music therapy allowed K to have some control over his environment. Honouring his desires, the music gently led K to his process of transformation allowing him to separate himself from this world to the next; his rite of passage.

Coda: comments from colleagues at Bethlehem Hospital about music therapy

The music therapist and the social worker have a number of common aims in a palliative care setting, whether in the home or hospice. It is our aim as part of a multi-disciplinary team to provide holistic care with respect for the individual's autonomy and choice, whilst providing support for carers, families and friends. Effective communication is central to this.

In palliative care, facilitating communication is a task for all team members. This interaction relies on the patient's ability and desire to participate in a highly verbal, and often taxing process. For those patients who are unable or uncomfortable with verbally expressing or exploring their emotions and needs, music therapy is especially effective. Whilst some of the music therapist's tools are common to those of the social worker (for example, life-reviews), it is often the creative use of music as a therapeutic tool that facilities effective communication of emotions and meaningful interaction between patients and their families and friends.

Often this experience becomes an important element when supporting the bereaved family.

Often the music therapy sessions taps into aspects of the patient's well being that other health professionals are unable to do. For the social worker, information attained during music therapy sessions becomes useful when planning the patient's ongoing care management.
(Kathryn Turner, BA. Dip. Ed., B.S.W. The University of Melbourne. Social Work Leader – Hospice Unit)

The final journey in life that leads ultimately to death is one that is often fraught with fears, anxieties and uncertainties. There our many challenges and hardships that are presented along this path which test our resolve and which present themselves in many forms. Climbing this mountain is perhaps the greatest challenge we face. Though, it does not need to be scaled alone. There are many that are prepared to be a companion.

There are many qualities which are required along this path that searches for resolution, harmony and peace.

What I am continually taught each day in caring for people who confront this ascent, is that it takes more strength to let go than it does to hold on. For some, this knowledge comes easily. For others, it is hard won.

Music therapy creates a bridge that leads to a vantage point from which people can experience the true meaning of strength, the key to their rite of passage. Music therapy is able to construct this bridge not only because of its craftsmen, but most importantly, due to the material of which it is built. Music!

I have been fortunate to witness on many occasions the power of music within a palliative care setting. Pharmaceuticals undoubtedly work for the many symptomatic issues which palliative care patients present. However, they often work by masking these symptoms so that they are no longer experienced. The gift of music takes a far more profound route. It enables self-growth, spiritual healing and a truly physical peacefulness.

The gift of music is one that touches all of us, enabling us to feel, experience, express, reflect and grow. It reaches inside and endeavours to find that melody which resonates uniquely within and to bring it into complete harmony and equilibrium.

The craft that allows the expression of the gift of music, music therapy, enables those who experience it the opportunity to explore the depths to find, as Bridgit Hogan writes earlier in this chapter, their 'path of acceptance and existential resolution' (p.70) as no other within the palliative care team can.

(Mark Cockayne, Coordinator – Hospice Home Care Program)

CHAPTER 6

Music Therapy in
Chronic Degenerative Illness

Reflecting the Dynamic Sense of Self

Wendy Magee

In recent years there has been an increasing interest in the area of palliative care for music therapists, largely stemming from the initial major contribution to the medical and music therapy literature about this work by Munro and Mount (Munro and Mount 1978). 'Palliative' as defined by the Concise Oxford Dictionary means 'anything used to alleviate pain, anxiety, etc.' With such a definition it could be considered therefore that music therapy is predominantly 'palliative' no matter what the client population. Within the music therapy literature, the term has largely come to be associated with individuals who are in hospice care and their support network. In more recent years, there has been an increasing interest in work with those living with HIV and AIDS (Bruscia 1991b, Bruscia 1995, Lee 1995; Lee 1996), including people who may not have the virus themselves but are affected by it in some way (Hartley 1994). This literature highlights the value of music therapy with individuals who are experiencing changes as a consequence of the illness whilst living with an unknown prognosis.

These issues, however, are also fundamental for individuals living with long term, incurable, degenerative illnesses that currently have no cure apart from symptomatic treatment. Individuals with Huntington's Disease, Multiple Sclerosis, Parkinson's Disease and Motor Neurone Disease live with conditions that are chronic, that is, the diseases are endured over many years. These diseases are also degenerative. Individuals experience many changes in different aspects of their well-being; physical, social and, with certain conditions, psychological. This causes the individual and their support network to have to constantly adapt to dynamically changing conditions. As one difficulty is acknowledged or solved, it changes its nature once again, or increases in complexity.

Little has been written in the music therapy literature about working with individuals with chronic neurological conditions and the implications for treatment of those conditions. Unlike work within the hospice setting, working with individuals living with degenerative neurological conditions can span over many years and many different stages of the illness. This paper will focus on music therapy with individuals with Huntington's Disease and Multiple Sclerosis, with whom the author has worked over a period of twelve years.

Chronic progressive neurological disease

Huntington's Disease (HD) is a chronic progressive hereditary disease affecting the central nervous system stemming from damage to the basal ganglia within the brain. It is most commonly characterised by large involuntary movements and abnormality of voluntary movements and gradual cognitive deterioration due to atrophying of the brain. Emotional disorders, behavioural problems and personality changes may be experienced, even to the extent of psychiatric symptoms such as schizophrenia and delusional disorders (Folstein 1989; Morris 1991). Speech is increasingly affected as the disease progresses and problems with cognition further influence aspects of communication such as initiation, spontaneity and the speed at which information is processed. Knowing and insight may be relatively well-preserved even into the most advanced stages of the illness (Shoulson 1990) The average age of onset is 36 to 45 years of age (Folstein 1989) and the degenerative process can be followed through early, middle and later stages. Studies examining the duration of the illness have yielded widely varying results, suggesting between 10 to 40 years' duration after onset (Harper 1991).

Multiple Sclerosis (MS) is a chronic progressive disease caused by the widespread breakdown of the covering of the nerve fibres throughout the brain and spinal cord, resulting in motor disturbances, sensory disturbances and changes in cognition (Walton 1977). Prognosis is highly variable between individuals and its aetiology is unknown. Although there is currently significant research investigating possible curative treatments, available treatment tends to be oriented to the relief of symptoms, or preventative in nature. Many people with MS experience cognitive dysfunction and recent research indicates that large numbers experience subcortical dementia (Mahler and Benson 1990). When combined with the severest possible symptoms of ataxia or paralysis impairing nearly all voluntary and functional movement, loss of speech, the inability to swallow, and extreme fatigue, the individual can experience self doubt, anxiety, and reduced self esteem (Randall 1982). It is individuals with such significant disabilities who will be referred to in this paper.

Songwriting in therapy

Certainly much of the literature concerning music therapy in HD and MS has focused on techniques used. This is largely due to the many problems with which the individuals present, and which the therapist must overcome in order to offer effective therapy. Music therapy with HD clients certainly has tended to focus on movement (Groom and Dawes 1985; Rainey Perry 1983), relaxation (Rainey Perry 1983), or speech production through singing (Erdonmez 1976; Hoskyns 1985; Rainey Perry 1983). Curtis (1987) and Dawes (1985a, 1985b) reflected the progressive nature of the illness through to the palliative stages using songs themes. Although clinical improvisation is described less frequently within the literature, I suggest that such a technique can help reveal and reflect important information about the individual's cognitive functioning within the early and middle stages of the disease process (Magee 1995a, 1995b). As the ability to verbally communicate deteriorates, the spontaneity and immediacy of improvising can offer an expressive outlet which is no longer available in words or movements. In my experience it is essential to monitor the appropriateness of methods employed considering cognitive changes, as these can impede the individual's music-making considerably. There remains however very little written about using music therapy with clients in the most advanced stages of the illness, or about working with clients over many years, which will be examined in one of the case studies included here.

Songwriting as a method of working with both MS and HD clients has been well documented. Brandt (1996) highlighted the role which songwriting can play in life review in the terminal stages of HD. O'Callaghan has argued the value of this technique with individuals with advanced MS in meeting physical, psycho-social and spiritual needs (O'Callaghan 1996a, 1996b and Chapter 3 in this book). Further techniques have been presented for working with individuals with advanced MS who showed considerable subcortical dementia and no functional movement, grounded in an understanding of individuals' cognitive abilities and maximising these using familiar music (O'Callaghan and Brown 1989; O'Callaghan and Turnbull 1987). This work offers valuable information for the therapist working with individuals whose disabilities would otherwise prevent them from engaging actively in the therapy process due to the severity of physical and cognitive disabilities. Lengdobler and Kiessling (1989) describe group therapy with more able MS patients exploring themes around disability, uncertainty, anxiety, depression, and loss of self esteem using minimally structured improvisations.

I have found in my clinical work, over a period of years, and research employing modified grounded theory analysis, that there are many issues working with clients with chronic degenerative illness that may be particular to this area of 'palliative' care. Certainly when living with chronic neurological illness, the individual may be faced with many years of increasing disability that changes gradually, but continually, over time. Unlike the individual in hospice care who may have a relatively short period of time to deal with very severe levels of disability and dependence, the expectation of long-term gradual deterioration is a reality for someone living with complex neuro-disability. Within music therapy sessions, with individuals living with chronic neuro-disability, I have observed a variety of methods of coping with uncertainty about changing needs and an unknown future. Research in progress with individuals with MS, is revealing that not only do individuals draw on certain coping mechanisms within their verbal and behavioural responses in music therapy sessions, but that such mechanisms are reflected also in the way individuals use and respond to music.

Individuals maintain what the author entitles a 'coping front' to mask less superficial or more difficult feelings and responses to particular events or their illness at large. In doing so, the individual manages to maintain on the outside what they perceive to be an acceptable side of themselves. Such coping mechanisms when they are expressed in verbal behaviour include stating rules, dismissing, projecting, keeping busy, masking and distracting. These are employed in situations where the individual feels less in control, under threat, refuses to accept their illness, or may be trying to find an explanatory framework for why they had acquired their illness. For example, an individual who may state verbally that they feel no negative consequence about losing their job, their home, and being isolated from their friends and family as a consequence of illness. In their choice of songs, however, they may choose songs that they associate with great sadness, loss and loneliness.

Within music therapy, the same coping mechanisms also influence how individuals talk about the music. Within clinical improvisations, individuals most often responded initially with concrete or literal representations of the music. Such representations included referring to improvisations as a conversation, counting the number of times an instrument was struck before moving onto another instrument, or moving from one specific instrument to the next to represent the register played by the therapist on her instrument. Although such concrete responses were initially attributed by the treatment team to cognitive deficits and difficulties interpreting abstract tasks, such as unfamiliar improvised music, clients' responses were observed to change over time. As the relationship with the therapist developed, individuals who previously had responded in a more concrete manner to improvisation were able to develop their musical responses and it was possible to gain a sense of what the improvisation represented to them through monitored post-session interviews.

It is possible that changes in cognition because of the disease process, rather than emotional responses, prevent some clients developing their musical material. The underlying cause must be assessed and interpreted objectively by the therapist if treatment is to optimise effect and meaning.

Using songs as coping strategies

The use of songs has been documented widely in the music therapy literature within palliative care, particularly examining the themes and lyrics of songs selected by the clients to communicate something personal as we have seen in earlier chapters. Within my work, I have identified that individuals request songs which represent particular emotional qualities or meanings. When maintaining a coping front, songs requested were linked with more positive emotional states such as 'happy', 'fun', 'cheerful' or 'positive', even when individual's behaviour and the themes contained within verbal material indicated that they felt far more vulnerable than such positive emotional states. Despite such use of music seeming superficial and the antithesis of the intended therapeutic goals, the importance in supporting individuals in their coping must be central to and direct the pace of therapy. Supporting clients in their coping in this way, is the only means to building a trusting relationship where the individual does not feel threatened, particularly if the relationship is to be a long term one.

More importantly, however, the individual who is maintaining a coping front through their words and behaviour, may indeed be lowering such a front in the way they use music to reach a state of barriers down. Such an emotional state is one where the individual is not only able to identify more difficult and painful feelings, but is able to relate such feelings to him or herself and acknowledge the effects the illness has had on his or her life.

Drawing on coping strategies was notably lowest immediately after songs which held great personal meaning to individuals. In relating to the emotional content of their song, individuals were able to move beyond the coping front to an emotional state where they could start to own the feelings they otherwise identified but masked outwardly. Understanding the theme or story of a song requested by the client is often the first step to acknowledgement within their coping process. It is the initial acknowledgement on a non-verbal musical level, which can then lead later to verbal exploration and acknowledgement, or exploration through improvisation.

Instrumental playing for those with neurological disability

Working with individuals who have advanced neurological disabilities presents many challenges for the therapist in finding instruments which are appropriate to meet a diverse range of needs. Instruments need to be safe for the uncontrolled nature of ataxic or choreic movements. They also need to be sensitive to the very small, weak or fatigued movements which typify the advanced forms of both HD and MS. Individuals with progressive degenerative conditions are often noted by their clinicians to monitor and measure even minor change closely. Although we may presume that the music therapy setting removes an individual from such pressures, individuals with chronic progressive illness have been observed to use their music therapy in this way.

I observed a phenomenon called illness monitoring through the involvement in music therapy. Individual patients monitor cognitive, vocal and physical changes that occur (Magee 1998). Through playing instruments within clinical improvisations, individuals monitored their physical abilities to manipulate instruments and control the sounds they produced. Such monitoring at times reduced the experience of improvising merely to a physical one, rather than one on any emotional level. Through singing familiar songs, individuals monitored their ability to recall the words to songs, and also their vocal production. Such comparisons were noted to occur within individuals, as well as between individuals who lived on the same residential ward or attended day care services with other patients with similar illnesses.

As the progressive nature of the illness takes its course, individuals have an ever-changing sense of self and identity which is gradual and long term. Such changes stem from gradually increasing disability, increasing dependence on others for even the smallest task, loss of skills or the opportunities to develop skills, reduced opportunities for achievement, and a very general sense of loss on many levels. Music therapy is able to challenge such an identity and facilitate development of a more able identity. Through the experience of improvisation, individuals reported that they had heightened experiences of ability, independence, skill, ownership, achievement and success (Magee 1998). Individuals reported feeling 'professional' and 'successful' in what they had achieved, and through developing the skills associated with music making, unmet hopes and dreams were stimulated leading to life review.

The patient as musician

When working with clients over many years, the therapist is able to gain an intimate knowledge of the individual as musician – what music in its essence represents and expresses for the individual. Such meaning is highly individual. Understanding the musical make-up of our clients involves knowing what pre-composed music represents to them as well as how they interact within a clinical improvisation. When working with clients in the advanced stages of neurological illness, there is a need for a model of music therapy where the client is able to be passive to a larger extent. Adopting a passive role does not imply that the patient is simply a non-participant listener but participant to the extent their abilities will allow. If the therapist is to continue working with the client into the terminal stages of their illness, working in such a way is essential. As physical and cognitive factors of the illness render the client's movements to become non-functional, arousal levels to become severely reduced, and ability to respond in an interactive way extremely limited, music continues to remain a 'way in'.

The following case studies will aim to highlight some of the points covered above. The first will examine the impact of music therapy on identity in a young man with advanced MS. The second will describe the changing application of music therapy with a woman who progressed from the middle to terminal stages of HD.

Chris

Chris was a man in his early thirties who received individual music therapy for a period of six months. He had advanced MS, having had a diagnosis for seven years. He was hospitalised 18 months earlier as he could no longer care for himself in his home. When seen for music therapy he was in a wheelchair, and had no functional movement in one of his arms. Although he had some voluntary movement in his other arm, this was severely ataxic which rendered it largely non-functional. He was dependent on others for all his personal needs. Although he could still speak, his speech was becoming slurred and difficult to understand at times. Neuropsychological assessments indicated that he was showing evidence of subcortical dementia, particularly affecting memory, learning, insight and abstract thought. His cognitive deficits exacerbated the emotional experience of his increasing dependence and disability, particularly as he was unable to reason through why he needed care in order to prevent his condition becoming more complicated medically.

Chris referred himself to music therapy on the grounds that he had previously played in rock bands and enjoyed being creative. Sessions were individual, weekly and lasted approximately 45 minutes. They were held in the music therapy room. He often arrived at sessions in an agitated and frustrated state. Within sessions he expressed many feelings verbally and musically about his increasing levels of dependence, disability, and overwhelming anger at his continual experience of loss. He quickly dismissed any difficult feelings he expressed by maintaining a front of indifference that seemed to be his way of coping. The focus of his music therapy became a place to explore his remaining abilities, challenge his disabled identity, and support him in his expression of the strong emotions with which he was struggling.

In the first ten sessions Chris's music within clinical improvisations consisted largely of playing an unfaltering loud pulse on selected drums and cymbals, showing little interactive response in his music to the therapist's music. He maintained continual eye contact with the therapist, which more resembled a glare. Immediately after improvisations, he often commented that he had been singing familiar songs to himself that he had been playing in his own mind. He made many comments about 'bashing' instruments and said that he felt unskilled. He attributed little musical sense to his own part in the improvisations. He made many temporal references to the musical abilities and skills he had possessed prior to his illness. He requested songs from the rock and popular repertoire which he identified as 'violent', 'raucous' or 'hippy'. He used such songs to maintain what he perceived to be a nonchalant front with the therapist. Overall his use of music within sessions was largely non-interactive and appeared emotionally deceptive.

A change in the therapeutic relationship occurred in session 10 when the therapist played a song which Chris had requested in a previous session but had not been found until this time. This song held many associative qualities for Chris which stretched back over 15 years. In his own words, the song symbolised a time when 'everything was possible and nothing was wrong with me'. His behavioural and emotional responses to this song were immediate and markedly different. The temporal and associative qualities of the song gave it great emotional meaning for Chris, and he started to allow his barriers down by acknowledging his illness and relating to the difficult feelings he had. Although he related his feelings verbally, it was the music through which the therapy relationship started to deepen. In future sessions he used this song to express his feelings musically at times when he could not acknowledge them verbally.

Within the clinical improvisations the relationship also started to develop. There began to be greater interaction within the musical components, and his playing became a little less organised, sparser, with less frequent occurrences of his relentless pulse. The meter changed from his relentless 4/4 to a more lilting 6/8. He also started to refer verbally to dramatic and emotionally expressive music from 19th and 20th century musical repertoire. His involvement in improvising, however, remained impeded by his physical fatigue and he expressed frustration that he could not play in the way he wished due to his ataxia. It appeared that his physical abilities limited the expressive qualities he wished to achieve in the music.

He arrived at session 18 in a highly emotional state related once more to his dependence on the nursing staff for all aspects of his care. The session consisted of three short, powerful improvisations. In discussing his feelings about the music afterwards he related the music back to the 'frustrating' events prior to the session, and stated that the music had represented someone 'who was in charge of everything'. He expressed having a heightened sense of ability within the music, and also feelings of success and achievement. He also reported that my 'aggressive' bass had matched his own aggressive beating of a drum.

Understanding the meaning of his special songs revealed musical and interpersonal elements which met him emotionally and helped him acknowledge the changes brought about by his illness. By building the trust in this way, he was able to explore these feelings further within improvisation. Although his physical and cognitive deterioration may prevent active music therapy at a future stage, I now had enough knowledge about the individual meaning of music to this man to apply a passive model if appropriate through the use of his particular songs.

Anna

Anna was a woman in her mid fifties with HD who had been hospitalised for nine years. Prior to the onset of her the disease 18 years ago, Anna led an extremely active life, having been a keen amateur instrumentalist and chorister. She had a great love of music which had played a major role in her life. Her music therapy spanned seven years which reflected different stages of her illness. Three different music therapists had been involved in her treatment, however the author has been involved in all stages except the individual period. Her case study also highlights the importance of the multidisciplinary team in meeting the complex needs of an individual with neuro-disability.

Anna was first referred for music therapy seven years earlier as part of a ward group run by the music therapist and a speech therapist over one year. Within this group, Anna was the most socially able, the most verbally communicative, and the most physically able member. At this time, she was still able to walk or stand with assistance, and in fact on one occasion she was able to dance with the author and one other person assisting. Her responses within weekly sessions were consistent. She tended to interact with staff rather than other participants, she sang and played to music within the group, became exuberant during music activities and exhibited a spontaneity in her music making. She was able to interact with other group members at this stage by watching, reaching out, and within brief musical interactions in which she could participate independently.

Following this group she received individual therapy for a period of a year. During this time, there was a marked deterioration in her verbal communication. She continued to be highly enthusiastic in her playing, although the purposefulness and meaning underlying her playing became difficult to interpret due to the large choreic movements that characterise the disease. Her musical material started to indicate some cognitive changes in her inability to imitate dynamics or rhythms given in the therapist's music, and difficulty with initiation of new musical material. Perseverative features were also reported in her playing, and verbally she became fixed on topics unrelated to the music. There was, however, an overwhelming sense of spontaneity and expression of humour about her music making which she sustained for long periods without tiring. The instruments she favoured were notably those with large surface areas and those sensitive to the touch, such as the cymbal, the bass xylophone and the wind chimes.

As her musical and verbal material in the individual therapy became directionless, and increasingly perseverative, participation in a group was recommended which she attended for the next two and half years. This was a very difficult time for her as she progressed into the advanced stages of the illness. Her movements became larger and more frequent, her positioning in her wheelchair became more difficult to maintain, this in turn considerably affecting her ability to play musical instruments and interact with others. Despite such, she remained 'exuberant' in her playing.

Within this group, four years ago, the spontaneity in her music continued much the same. Her responses, however, became more delayed and she had great difficulty physically manipulating instruments that she had previously held without difficulty.

With the arrival of a new seating system, her positioning was improved, which increased her alertness, enhanced her physical abilities, and generally increased her responses. As time progressed, her responses became generally slower and more delayed. She became less aware, showing less initiative. This increased her isolation within the group. Adaptations to instruments, which were previously played successfully, needed to be continually assessed as they started to prove less effective. Her responses indicated that she was not comprehending verbal instructions effectively. Despite such deterioration, she continued to participate spontaneously and exuberantly within musical activities. Vocalising became increasingly important, and she started to improvise vocally and spontaneously in immediate response when I played the flute.

Two years ago she progressed into what was considered to be the 'terminal' stages of the illness. This stage has lasted much longer than those caring for her expected. Too frail, and difficult to arouse, to be involved in any active therapy, the multidisciplinary team questioned her involvement in a music therapy group. Her responses within such, showed increased arousal, an awareness of my words and music, and she made attempts to communicate verbally. At this stage, her involuntary vocalisations were nearly constant, causing her voluntary vocalisations to be difficult to interpret. However her responses to certain musical stimuli, such as the flute, continued to elicit high falsetto vocalisations. These differed markedly in quality from the lower guttural vocal sounds she made involuntarily and on attempting to speak and occurred only during musical tasks. In this way, her awareness and intention could be confirmed. Her movements were no longer the large choreic ones more typical of the mid to late stages of the illness, but were now small, constant tremors. She was no longer able to choose instruments nor play them in any active way. This meant that her participation needed to be as an active listener or, when she felt able, on a vocal level. Drawing from my knowledge of Anna's favourite songs, I used techniques drawing on song choices covering a variety of moods and tempi within the selection offered. Anna was then able to play an active part in the group, express something about her mood and have it met in the music. Although individual therapy was considered at this point, it was thought that the group setting made less demands on her as she could respond as and when she was able to. The clinical team felt that Anna's death was near.

Due to changes within the hospital six months ago, it was necessary to wind the group down, and there was to be a new music therapist working on the ward. Within one of the last groups, Anna was highly responsive and interactive in her attempts to verbally communicate. She was offered a choice of two favourite songs from which to choose. Prior to the group I had planned to offer only 'brighter' songs due to Anna's frail state. I have often questioned why I considered doing this, and how much my own fear of Anna using music to express her feelings played a part. It was evidently a sensitive situation, and I was concerned that Anna's wishes or choices should not misconstrued by myself in any way. Within the session however, she was more alert and communicative than usual, which caused me to re-evaluate my decision. It was with some hesitation that I offered within the choice of songs one of her favourite songs by The Carpenters entitled 'Yesterday Once More', The words of this song embody reflections about change, loss, sadness, and coping with adversity. The lyrics of this song specifically refer to the way in which the temporal and associative properties contained within favourite love songs stimulate intense emotional states.

Anna in fact chose this song by clearly stating its title, and whilst it was being played, sang as many of the words as she could, more clearly and loudly than she had sung in the previous months. My own emotional reactions were strong, as I realised that my musical and therapeutic relationship with this woman were coming to an end. Although I was not able to sing all the words myself, Anna could be heard singing clearly, particularly the title of the song.

Her immediate responses afterwards were 'Wonderful song' and a smile. The thematic and lyrical content of the song expressed in many ways, both verbally and musically, sentiments and thoughts which she had no other means of expressing directly and as independently. It is also believed that her choice of this song rather than a 'brighter' song was specifically for such a purpose. In this way, she was using songs as a way of reviewing her life and expressing her feelings about her approaching death.

Coda

Anna chose not to continue with music therapy with a different therapist. She has lived longer than many of us caring for her thought she would. I feel I said my good-bye within the musical relationship with the playing of her song. Having worked with such a personal and intimate medium as music for so many years with an individual, I question whether I would have been able to continue offering her real support within music, or whether my own feelings would have hampered me from really meeting her within the music, as had started to happen at the end of our therapy relationship.

Acknowledgements

The author would like to acknowledge the clinical work of previous therapy colleagues Rosie Monahan and Cathy Durham in the second case study, and also of multidisiplinary colleagues at the Royal Hospital for Neuro-disability, London which received a proportion of its funding from the NHS Executive. The views expressed in this publication are those of the author and not necessarily those of the NHS Executive. Acknowledgements is made also of the supervision given by Dr Jane Davidson in the research material and the support of the John Ellerman Foundation and the Living Again Trust.

CHAPTER 7

Music

A Means of Comfort

Susan Weber

On the final evening, December 4, family and friends gathered around Mozart in Vienna to sing selections from the unfinished Requiem. Only seven stanzas of the 'Lacrimosa' were completed, and Mozart began to sing the alto part, imitating the trumpets by puffing out his cheeks. 'Here is my death song,' he said, invigorated by the music...

Shortly after midnight, Mozart died. On his deathbed, the child prodigy who had been bathed in music while still in the womb and the composer who could channel heaven-sent concertos and symphonies asked to be surrounded by music and singing. (Campbell 1997, pp.216–217)

The Johannes Hospiz d. Barmherzigen Brüder, in Munich, was opened in 1991. The Hospice was built as a model project for a palliative station in Bavaria for those suffering with malignant diseases and in the terminal phase of AIDS. It has 25 beds in single and double-rooms. The primary intention of all working in the hospice is to maintain the patient's time as free from pain and suffering as possible. (Grenzel, Binzack and *Hospizeinrichtung* 1995).

Great care has been given to offer a warm and caring environment for the patients. There is a high ratio of personal to patients – 1.2 nurses per patient. The building is situated within a park and has rooms that let in as much light as possible; slanted windows that allow the patients to look up into the trees; walls with gentle colours, wooden floors and beds; and guest-rooms for family members to spend the night. Even the diet is planned carefully to be both nutritious and appetising.

In 1997, the Johannes Hospice admitted 409 patients. Their ages ranged from 25 to 95 years, the average being 60. Two hundred and ninety one passed on in the hospice and 118 were released (returning home to die or going on to nursing homes); 376 were patients suffering with cancer, 9 were infected with HIV and 24 had other diseases. The average stay was 14 days.

I work within this environment twice a week as a music therapist. There is no formal system for introducing me to my patients. Because of the high turn over rate, I normally check which of my patients is still there and then ask the staff whom they feel I should see or who has asked to see me. Just as often members of staff, from the Directing Physician down to the cleaning personnel, approach me when I arrive and request that I see specific patients.

Music in the hospice

Although there are numerous aspects of music therapy in hospice work, I would like to discuss here what I have found to be the most helpful and meaningful uses for music in this particular house.

As a psychologist, I am often asked why I also choose to work as a music therapist. On the one hand, my patients often feel that they have so much unfilled time each day and on the other hand, time is no longer an available luxury. Some of this time can be filled with music and turned into quality time (O'Callaghan 1993).

Music's ability as a tool for communication has long been established (Hodges and Haack 1996). There is usually no time left for deep problem solving and music allows me to establish a quick rapport. This non-verbal communication can give my patents a sense of 'belonging' and trust, even if it is only temporary (Lochner and Stevenson 1987). In addition, music acts as a non-verbal catalyst of our feelings, evoking an emotional response, releasing material stored in our memories and facilitating the expression of feelings that are pleasant or those which we have buried because they were too difficult to deal with (Kenny 1982). Music allows results which might otherwise take weeks with normal psychotherapy and is a healing tool that affects people of every age and background.

Perhaps I am a shy psychologist, but I notice how much more relaxed I am when I ask a patient what music they would like to hear, play themselves or what I can play for them than when I am in my psychologist role. Most people are more willing to open up and discuss music with me than psychology. A relationship can be built on something positive that has nothing to do with their illness (Nolan 1992). They need warmth and friendship, too (Saunders 1965). Simply enjoying music together is a gift for both of us.

I am also often asked what place music has within all of the intensive care the hospice offers.

As a musician the reasons seem simple to me – music can restore a normal part of life to a patient. It has accompanied us life-long, even if unconsciously. Our music is a reflection of our period of time, personal and global and is symbolic for our experiences, ideas, behaviours and philosophies of life. It is a mirror of our worlds – past, present and future – our personal life story (Storr 1992).

I have yet to meet anyone who has led a life without music whether they were sung to as a baby, went dancing as a young person, chose music for their wedding, or sang to their own children. And always we have had our favourite music to hear, sing or play.

Music is an art form. An early Cluniac abbot wrote that the maintenance, cultivation and refinement of beauty is one way to encounter the face of the Divine (Schroeder Sheker 1993). We humans have a need for the beautiful and the Divine. The aesthetic enjoyment of music satisfies these needs with the dying – perhaps in a way no other art form can.

Music enhances our worlds, let's us forget our stress, and enervates us, contributing greatly to our sense of physical, emotional and spiritual well-being. These matters are still or even more important when we are going through the death process. Based on these reasons, it would seem illogical not to use music with the dying.

There are many ways that I use music with my patients. I begin by asking a patient if he or she would like some of their favourite music to listen to on a cassette player (Munro 1984). If the hospice doesn't have it, I try and find the tape for them (in this way our cassette collection has grown). This is an easy place to start. Although many people say, 'I am not musical' or 'I do not understand anything about music', they still want to listen to it. Since most of our patients are very ill and close to dying, they do not have the physical strength to play an instrument themselves. They also have a lot to cope with and don't need any big new projects. This listening provides an element of safety and seems to provide the support and distance necessary to sometimes broach frightening or otherwise difficult topics.

The next time I see them, they often tell me how much they love listening to the music. They are also often eager to explain why they like it, when and how it was important to them, and if they had played it themselves. I have repeatedly experienced patients quickly sharing their life stories through the music they were listening to or I was playing for them. It was as if the music had opened up a deep desire and a way to share these experiences. For example, I no longer know how many times I have played German folk songs and had a patient start singing along or share the happy memories of their family singing while they were all still together. These older people grew up singing. For a generation that lost so much, sometimes those early memories of song are their happiest or reflect a time 'before everything became so difficult'. Most of them went through wars, prison camps, were perpetrators or victims and never had any concrete means of working through so much horror. Music can open a door to these very painful experiences that many of them have never discussed and are often desperate to find some relief either from real or imagined guilt and terrible personal suffering. I feel that these are some of my most important moments in helping people heal old wounds, find their spiritual resources and die easier.

On the other hand, if I have a sense that a patient wants to talk and doesn't know where to begin, I ask some easy questions: 'What made you choose that music?' 'Why do you like it?' 'When did you first hear it?' 'Did you ever play it yourself?' I really want to know because the answers are always interesting and they share so much – meaningful parts of their lives without me having been overly intrusive. And some patients say, 'No thank you. I just want to be quiet.'

Helping patients relax is also a high priority in my work. Few patients arrive at the hospice in a relaxed state. They have just taken their last trip and are usually tense, emotionally overloaded, frightened, depressed and physically exhausted (Whittall 1989).

I sometimes see them very soon after their arrival, especially if they are alone, or a day or two later. They are very surprised by my appearance and even more surprised when I push a piano into the room. Many are too sick or weak to request favourite music and just nod when I ask them if they would like me to play for them. I try to create an oasis of peace and harmony. I don't ask them any questions. I just play the piano or a small Veeh harp,[1] usually gentle and tender music. This is a time when they don't have to do anything except lie back and lean on the music. It is a neutral medium but a familiar

---

[1]   Veeh, Hermann, Harfenbauer. Ochsenfürtenstr. 32, 97258 Guelchsheim

one, offering support with a definite structure and rhythm, melody and harmony. I start with slow music of about 60 beats and slow it down to around 50 beats – if the patient feels comfortable with this. Although the slower rhythm has a more effective relaxing effect, not everyone can immediately handle it and some people have to be led into it. I have also asked a composer friend to write gentle music that I can play ever slower,[2] because many pieces starts to fall apart if they are played so much slower than the composer intended. My patients seem to prefer structured compositions rather than pure improvisation. Some patients ask that I repeat one piece over and over – the repetition helps them fall asleep. This kind of music is also a help for patients experiencing insomnia, respiratory and neurological problems.

I have been and still am collecting gentle music with lovely melodies which offer emotional support. However, it is not always so easy to find gentle music that is not also sad and/or melancholy. Perhaps sadness is more accepted than tenderness in this society. If patients need to express their sadness, and they often do, I try to also help them reconnect to their own tender feelings. I sense that this can be a beginning of the process of forgiveness and further the inner healing process.

The music will support them and they start to let down quicker, relax and eventually express some of their emotions and/or concerns. If they want – they have someone to talk to. They often cry silently and then sleep. Many times, we haven't spoken much, but they have found some relief.

On another day it may seem appropriate to ease the music into a more lively vein, the rhythmic stimuli stir up muscular tensions which can be released through physical activity. In other words, a foot starts to tap a little or a hand moves or the patient maybe smiles a little. All of this can help to pull the patient out of his morbid preoccupation with himself, directing his attention towards things and events around him. By feeling more life and having some fun, a patient may become more willing to start changing negative attitudes and perhaps make some deeper contact with his family.

Even when my patients are very weak, they can still be agitated or trying to resolve problems internally. Playing soothing music is often a big aid in helping them quiet down and start dealing with difficult issues. Here again,

2   Anderle, Martin Christian, 'Melodies of Peace.' Grünhütlstr. 8, D 86911 Diessen

some patients ask me to repeat the same music over and over, saying it 'helps them think things through'.

Music can also be effective in calming the agitated patient who is no longer alert, non-responsive or comatose. I have found singing softly to be effective here because of the effect of the human voice and it is so easy to entrain with the patient's breathing, reflecting his breathing in the music so that in a way, the two of us are singing together. I can then gradually slow the tempo down or keep it very steady. In this way, I have also awakened several comatose patients.

We sometimes have patients arriving who have spent a long time on an intensive care unit which is an extremely loud and hectic place. In addition to the general quiet atmosphere of our hospice, this kind of music and/or singing wraps them in peace and security and restores some serenity.

Pain management

Pain management is a major part of hospice care. It is a priority that all patients are relieved of their pain. We also have patients who are here only to receive a morphium pump and are able to go home and enjoy extra months with a relatively good quality of life. They are usually with us about two weeks and are often stronger and in better shape than our other patients. Music can help them through distraction, alteration of mood, and promoting relaxation (Magill Levreault 1993). Helping with relaxation and calming and sedative music can again be a valuable aid here. Although the pain cannot be controlled with music alone, patients are glad to use music to help themselves relax and love to be 'played to sleep'. Many of them like to play the harp and actively participate in music making. Although they know they only have a few months left, dying isn't dead. Making music lets them be creative and creativity is life-giving and life-enhancing (Olofsson 1995).

The Veeh harp has proven very appropriate for my Hospice work with these patients as one can play familiar melodies without reading music. It only weighs two and one half kilos, is easy to handle and the patients enjoy the gentle sound. Although we do have some percussion instruments, they are hardly used with the exception of the ocean drum. Most of our patients are either not interested or find them too strenuous.

Family and friends

The hospice staff is also very concerned and caring about family members and close friends of the dying. They have also been suffering, trying to manage a family alone, are weary, frightened, trying to deal with powerful emotions and need support themselves (Stedeford 1981). I try also to include them in some of the musical activities where possible.

For example, sometimes when I am with a patient, their wife or husband will join us. I play the music they have enjoyed together, such as songs that were popular when they first met, were beginning their relationship and the music they have enjoyed together over the years. The patient and/or the family member often later tell me it was just nice to sit quietly and listen together. They never had much time to 'just sit and listen'. If we have time, we put together a musical cassette of their favourite music for the surviving spouse to keep.

Not all relationships have been harmonious and patients also relate that the music and the associated memories can make it easier for them to start talking to each other.

Often the female patients are very concerned that their husbands come and don't know what to do. They are relieved to have the music as it keeps them occupied and calms them down, at least while I am playing. (Female spouses seem to handle the dying process better than males.) Family members can also be very disruptive by continuously talking, roaming around etc. or they simply do not want me there. In these cases, I try and find a time when I will be alone with the patient. On the other hand, there are times when I feel I am playing more to comfort the family member than the patient. I often make tapes for family members to use at home for their own relaxation.

When I am working with confused patients, those with short term memory lapse, dementia or loss of speech, it is of deep meaning for the family to see them start to react, trying to speak and sing with me. It is a reminder that the 'person' is still there, even if the brain is no longer functioning as it once was. If the family wishes, I find the music and lyrics that they have sung and we sing together with the patient.

As stated, when patients have been so agitated, it is reassuring for the family to see them settle down to the music and this allows them to find their own peace as they are usually upset and feeling helpless. It is again a comfort and relief for the family when a patient comes out of a coma. They have one or more opportunities to talk with the patient and say 'good-bye' even when the patient can no longer speak.

As a patient gets closer to death, the music becomes simpler – like a mother singing lullabies. I actually do use a book of lullabies. Although patients may have loved listening to Mozart or similar music when they first arrived, for many it has become too complicated. I play a lot of English, Irish, Scottish and Welsh folk songs because of their gentleness and simple melodies. The patients and families love them. This is a time when I also sing more. When patients were stronger, we have often sung them together and I often accompany these songs with the Veeh harp.

Singing 'good-bye'

When a patient is alone or the family request it, I play while the patient is dying, when possible up to and during his death. Hearing is the sensory organ which usually functions until the end (Tomatis 1996) so I know they can still hear me, even when they can no longer see or speak. I feel that whatever may be happening 'on the other side', it is important that the patient feel the presence of someone here with them – that they are not alone. (This is also hospice policy.) I play sacred music, or music I know had a particular meaning for the patient, or music that has a particular meaning for me. I feel that this is a great privilege. Sometimes I play the piano or harp, and sometimes I just sit with them and sing 'good-bye'. We have often become friends and I want them to feel my care and love accompanying them on 'this side'. I can think of nothing more appropriate for me to give them than the music we have shared together.

At other times, I have played for the family after the death to allow them to calm down and find peace before going home.

Finally, it happens that the family asks what music I was playing or what the patient's favourite music was and we arrange the music for the funeral together.

Case study 1

Herr L was 50 years old and suffering from prostate cancer. When I first started working with him, he had brain metastases which gradually worsened causing blindness, but did not affect his lucidity. He had been a factory worker at BMW, the German automobile maker. The staff asked me to see him as he had reported an interest in music.

When I visited him initially, he was very reticent and shy, as I was. At this time, the piano had not yet arrived in the hospice and so I showed him the Veeh harp and he played it a little. However, he didn't show much interest and his sight was starting to fail. I asked him if I could bring him some tapes of his favourite music. The change was very dramatic. He immediately lit up and leaned towards me. He told me that music had been his whole life and that he had been unable to get any higher education because he had to support the younger members of his family. No one at home had ever understood his deep love of music. He had been an avid concert and opera-goer, often standing, as that was all he could afford. He was delighted to finally have someone to talk about music with. It turned out that we had been in many of the same concerts and opera performances. He then asked me to bring him music he didn't know so he could learn something new. It developed into our game. The only thing I ever found that he was unfamiliar with was some piano music by Louis Gottschalk. As he completely lost his sight, I also started reading to him from a book of personal reminisces by famous musicians from Karl Böhm to Karajan and other biographies of musicians. We had long discussions about how we experienced them through reading the text out loud. I then started finding the recordings they mentioned so he could listen to those too. We did this for six weeks. The night before he passed on, there was a live harp concert in the hospice. I did not want him to have to go to another concert alone and sat with him in his room. He was too weak to sit up or talk but just held on to my hand. He died the next morning.

My work with Herr L was one of the most memorable times I experienced with a patient. I was touched to share this precious, hidden part of his life. He lived much longer than anyone had expected. The staff and I felt that in addition to finally being able to share his love of music, he was finally getting the love, attention and appreciation he had never had from all of us. And he soaked it up for as long as he could.

Case study 2

Frau K was a psychologist in her late fifties suffering from breast cancer. She was initially in the hospice for pain control and very mobile. She saw me tuning the harp and asked what it was. I showed it to her and she played it at once. I left it with her along with all the music I had. The next time I saw her, I suggested we play together. (The hospice has 2 harps for this purpose.) We played together for a month. It was the first instrument she had ever played. She had also been a real caregiver for her patients and her husband and told me it was one of the few times that she had time for herself to do what she wanted and had the time to try something new. I transcribed more music for us as we were getting bored with the simple duets and she wanted to see how 'good' we could get. A nurse or two often joined us for a few minutes to listen and have some fun with us. She was delighted to be able to play for others. As I was also a psychologist, we often moaned, groaned and laughed about all our similar professional experiences. She was normally very reticent and I do not think she would have opened up with me so quickly, or I with her, if we hadn't first been making music together. She returned home for several weeks and returned to the hospice, dying very unexpectedly.

Coda

For our hospice patients, who have often suffered so much, music brings them something beautiful. So many sick and older people have been very alone and music can pull them out of their isolation and make it easier to share their concerns and joys. Music helps them calm down and face personal issues that are not always so pleasant. I also try and make our time together, the music we listen to and I play, very personal and individual for them – something that is theirs alone. It can also be something special shared with family members. Several people have told me how they often remember later those happy hours we had together.

Music often fills a spiritual need or reconnects them to their own spirituality, reopening a door that had been closed for a long time. It is not unusual for patients to ask me to pray with them after we have been sharing music.

For myself, making music is simple and uncomplicated, and something very intimate. Music is also my therapy, acting as a buffer for some of the very difficult and painful things I witness, and offers me a vehicle to express and deal with my own feelings and restore my emotional equilibrium.

I am convinced that music plays a distinctive and valuable role in a palliative care program. It is very beautiful and special, unmatched in its ability to touch, move and affect us. I can no longer imagine working without it.

CHAPTER 8

Music Therapists' Personal Reflections on Working with Those Who Are Living with HIV/AIDS

Nigel Alan Hartley

Let me tell you… there is something very odd indeed about this music of yours. A manifestation of the highest energy – not at all abstract, but without an object, energy in a void, in pure ether – where else in the universe does such a thing appear?…But here you have it, such music is energy itself, yet not as idea, rather in its actuality. I call your attention to the fact that this is almost the definition of God… (Mann 1949, p.78)

Prelude

Over the last twenty years, the Human Immunodeficiency Virus (HIV) has become a major health care challenge. AIDS is one of the major health epidemics of our time and however we choose to deal with it – whether we ignore it, whether we accept it and then turn a blind eye to it, or whether we persecute those who are living with it, or whether we involve ourselves in the direct care of those who are affected by it – we are all influenced by its presence. Lives are changed because of it. A time has come – as predicted in the early eighties – when the majority of us will know, directly or indirectly, someone who is living with, or who has lived with the virus.

Since the first appearances of the virus almost eighteen years ago, groups of people have come together and responded to the challenge in various ways. London Lighthouse – the United Kingdom's first major residential and support centre for those living with HIV/AIDS – is now well into its twelfth year. It is here, over the past five years or so, that I have worked as a music therapist with adults, families and children who have been affected by the virus. The unique story of Lighthouse – how it came about amidst strong reaction from the local community – is well documented (Cantacuzino 1993; Spence 1996).

The institution's vision statement at the Lighthouse outlines the philosophy of the project that is to tackle the challenges faced by people affected by HIV and AIDS. Its main aims and commitments are as follows:

- To provide high-quality care and support, in centres and people's homes, to empower people with HIV and AIDS to live and die well.

- To promote the changing attitudes to HIV and AIDS and to help make sure good public policies and services for affected people are developed.

- To make sure that people living with HIV and AIDS are central to the organisation, so they can influence policies, develop services and actively contribute to the decision-making process.

- To create safe and welcoming environments which offer time and space to meet the needs of the service users, carers, paid and unpaid staff and visitors.

- To challenge the denial of death – to bring the issue of death into the open and recognise that it is part of life and living.

- To challenge oppression, discrimination and prejudice, promote equal opportunities and to speak up for social justice.

Lighthouse is indeed a special place. Reactions of visitors are always telling. After a visit there a few years ago, an American music therapist wrote to me: 'It's one of those rare places where it's clear from the moment you enter the building the place and the people in it are there for a common reason. The air is thick with passion, commitment, acceptance, and people just getting on with their lives…'

People who have become infected with HIV have reacted to it differently in terms of physical and emotional manifestations – it is a complex illness. For those attempting to provide a cure, this has made it difficult to pinpoint the virus in any concrete way. Over the years, the HIV community has lived through intense periods of experiencing fear, loss, anger, desolation, isolation, guilt and unworthiness. The strength of an institution such as Lighthouse has been, and continues to be, that it aims to hold, support and enable those who are living through such unbearable suffering to '...look death in the eye whilst living life to the full...' (Spence 1996, p.139). It has also given those who are living with HIV/AIDS a voice. This voice is listened to with respect, offering those affected by the virus a strong sense of being heard and acknowledged.

As music therapists, we are influenced by the institutions within which we work. At Lighthouse, where the clientele are given involvement and influence, situations will not be tolerated where the aim of one person is solely to change another. Therapy will not work, therefore, if the therapist sets out to change his patient. 'Being with' as opposed to 'being in control of', and 'accepting' as opposed to 'working for change' are expected and belong to the patient by right. Of course change occurs, but it is not the major focus. Therapist and patient move together on a journey through the unknown – discovery, encounter and adventure providing a heart to the work.

At present, we live through a period of immense hope with current developments in new drug combinations offering a time when people are not only living longer, but are living healthily for longer. We are reminded, however, not to become too complacent. Those who are not responding to the new treatments must not be forgotten, and the current crisis in developing countries must continue to be ever present in our minds.

Over the years, Lighthouse has managed a formidable task. On one hand, it has remained true to its vision, never forgetting why it is there. On the other, it has moved constantly, changing from an organisation where a high percentage of service users are gay men into one that can meet the needs of the women, children, and heterosexual men who have become infected.

In his book *On Watch – Views from the Lighthouse* (1996), Spence explores the subject of learning from new experiences. In the following passage, he talks about how the organisation dealt with the death of a member of staff:

> ...his coffin was brought through the front door and laid down in reception. Many members of staff had gathered in welcome and flowers were laid...With his return, reality could at last sink in and people began to grieve, arms wrapped round one another for support. Even though we are accustomed to death at Lighthouse, I had never before seen the organisation intuitively dealing with its loss in such a public manner. I remember looking out beyond the circle of mourners and noticing that others were going abut their business in the usual way, apparently unconcerned by the scene round the coffin. People were everywhere,

coming to eat in the cafe, passing through to a training course, delivering packages at reception, arriving to call on residents. At this moment I understood in a new way that part of our vision statement which affirms that death and dying are central to life and living, that these issues need bringing out into the open. Here were life and death, side by side, in healthy balance... Lighthouse never felt safer...it was a glimpse of what is possible...(p.138)

Music and music therapy have played an important part at Lighthouse over the years. Colin Lee had initiated the inclusion of music therapy within the institutions therapeutic programme for his doctoral research and his pioneering work is well documented (Lee 1989, Lee 1992, Lee 1996). When I began, early in 1993, there had been no music therapy for almost two years. My place had been made secure by a secondment from the Nordoff-Robbins Music Therapy Centre in London. I began working one afternoon a week changing to a full day six months later. Nordoff-Robbins provided the salary, whilst Lighthouse bought instruments and provided a space to work. This space, The Ian McKellan Hall, is a significant room. Not only does it house music therapy but also funerals, meetings, conferences, fund-raising events and concerts. Most of my work still takes place here, although occasionally I work on the Residential Unit with those who are too sick to come to the hall. Referrals come from a mixture of sources; from other colleagues – doctors, nurses, other therapists and volunteers – and also outside organisations such as general medical practitioners (GPs) and psychiatrists. The majority of patients make choices themselves, the largest group of people that I work with are self-referred.

Writing

So why does our writing matter, again? they ask.

Because of the spirit, I say. Because of the heart. Writing and reading decrease our sense of isolation... It's like singing on a boat during a terrible storm at sea. You can't stop the raging storm, but singing can change the hearts and spirits of the people who are together on that ship. (Spence 1996, p.16)

I have the impression in the music therapy world, that unless we write about our work we are not taken seriously. I have never wanted to write just for the sake of it. To be honest, writing about music scares me somewhat. I sit here surrounded by audio tapes of individual and group music therapy sessions created together with patients at Lighthouse over the years. Every now and again I take one out and listen to part of it; memories of people, most of whom now dead, come instantly to mind. I am re-reminded that although these musical portraits, these musical journeys can be recounted factually, there is something at the centre of musical improvisation that defies verbal interpretation.

The word 'journey' is often given to an individual process which leads towards death. Accompanying the person on that journey is another word that is regularly used to describe the part played by the professional, be it therapist, doctor, nurse, befriender or chaplain. Although I have been part of many peoples journey, I find that I must not lose sense of my own. My own journey as a music therapist working in this area is full of vivid memories and moments of deep experience, all of which help me towards a clearer understanding of the work. The irony here is the impossibility of verbalising the understanding. This lies at the heart of my fear of writing about the work, 'What if it's not what I mean?'

In a conversation with Christopher Spence, Founder Director of London Lighthouse, he once said to me: 'Someone is always going to criticise what you say; you may as well be criticised for speaking the truth!'

So I attempt to write about what I really believe, part of which is that musical experience cannot be successfully explained. In writing about what goes on around musical experience, problems occur, for then we are removing ourselves from the act of creating music and attempting to make sense of it in retrospect. Often, when talking after the event with patients, all sense of the experience itself gets lost and the exercise becomes impossible. However, from time to time, it is what the patients have said about the experience of improvising music that has inspired me towards a clearer and deeper understanding.

Of course, when listening to what the patient says about the musical experience, we have the added problems of how we listen to, and respond to, their verbal comments. When working as a counsellor, my supervisor once helped me with a difficult situation. I was finding it impossible to work out what a client meant by what they were saying, to the point where I was ceasing to hear what it was she was actually saying at all. She said: 'Listen to what the person is saying – not to what you think they are saying! Listen to what is said – not to what you think might be missing! There is much to be learned here...' So, if I listen to what a person is saying now about a musical experience, straightforwardly, clearly and honestly, I know that there is much to be learned.

What follows are a series of experiences, thoughts and reminiscences drawn from my time at Lighthouse. Included within these are verbal comments – when appropriate – from particular patients. When in doubt just read the words – do not interpret them.[1] When discussing, or playing audio/video recordings of patients' work in music therapy, we must do so with the utmost respect. Here are people, more often than not, in vulnerable situations. Even though permission to use this material has always been given, I entrust their words and stories to your care.

> …The critics will say of this effusion that it isn't what I said it would be…and that it has too many irrelevancies, instant value judgements on music, too little 'pulling my socks up' about AIDS. In answer I can only echo the Grand Old Man Vaughan Williams, who said after the indifferent reception given to the ninth symphony, 'It was what I meant.' It has always been what I meant. (Rees 1991, p.170)

Life and death

> It is right it should be so
> Man was made for Joy and Woe,
> and when this we rightly know,
> through the world we safely go.
> Joy and woe are woven fine,
> a clothing for the soul divine,
> under every grief and pine
> runs a joy with silken twine.
>
> (William Blake's *Auguries of Innocence,* lines 55–60)

There is a school of thought that believes that most art is borne out of suffering. The image of the suffering artist producing works of staggering beauty is nothing new – artists, such as Van Gogh, and musicians, such as Rachmaninov, are immediately brought to mind. Suffering, with regard to dying, is also something that is widely written about (Byock 1994; Fiddes

---

1   Editor's note: This is impossible to achieve, as understanding is the interpretation of what is being read. What the author intends is that we take at face value what the patient has to say and respect what it is that he or she says.

1988; Gregory 1994). In my experience of working with those who are facing death, it is not so much the fear of death itself that plays a prominent role but the fear of the journey towards death which becomes the major focus – 'Why do I have to go through such pain, such suffering?'

In life, death is a given – none of us will escape this – even though the majority of people will choose not to think about it at a deep level until faced with a crisis. Lighthouse acknowledges that although people die from AIDS related illnesses, people can also be enabled to live with both HIV and AIDS. Consequently, the infection is seen from a different angle, there is potential for it to become slightly more bearable. From this perspective, people are living with HIV and not dying with it.

Many of those I have worked with talk about the fact that when given the diagnosis of HIV positive, a part of themselves dies. Being creative in music offers the potential for patient and therapist to be fully alive together. Blake's references to joy and woe are significant here. Joy and woe must be as inseparable as life and death. Out of woe comes joy, out of suffering comes beauty, and out of the reality of death comes a deeper understanding of life. This being the case, out of the experience of being fully alive in music must come a new comprehension of death and the dying process.

James

James, an HIV positive man in his thirties describes how music therapy affected him:

Music therapy helped to break down the barriers after my diagnosis as HIV positive. It offered me the chance, and the challenge, to set out on a previously unattempted journey of creative self-exploration at the moment I could have retreated into passivity and despair. Music is so big, it always has room, and a vocabulary, for whatever one wants to express. Yet the silence it incorporates and out of which it grows, is acutely charged with the potential for listening and being heard. During the sessions I never felt my personality, or my situation, being diminished by the imposition of a simplistic methodology. Sometimes I had to overcome the fear of making a self-exposing gesture; but was always rewarded with the grace of meaningful response. By means of the journey, with the music therapist as a constant support and companion, I became the creator, but also the sharer, of beauty. I am, then, no longer surprised by people relating their experiences of improvising music during music therapy sessions to an improved quality of life – I feel so much better, I don't know where the energy comes from are common reactions. Some HIV positive patients talk about how a new understanding of life has been gained from the experience of creating music during therapy sessions.

Mario

Mario was a patient with whom I worked over a period of three months before he died. He was in his sixties and had recently become a grandfather. The weekly sessions were full of a rich variety of music and often he would improvise huge operatic arias which I would accompany from the piano. These arias would often be in Italian and, although I rarely understood the verbal content, I matched the intensity of the melodic contour and the harmonic direction of his vocal lines. Physically he was ill and very weak. Both myself and my colleagues were surprised by the enormous energy and commitment that manifested itself in the music that we improvised. During one of our final sessions together, he spoke the following words:

> You know, my body is fading away by the day – the outside of me is dying; when were improvising the focus is on the inside – the inside of me is living, and when we play it grows and expands… We have two very clear things; I refer to these as your music and my music. Initially we are separate, and then, almost always, something special happens. Then what we have is what I would call our music. Here, we are totally one, totally equal – in balance. During these times there is no illness, I am completely well; in fact I never felt so alive!

Both James and Mario make important statements. For James, the experience of improvising music brought him out of an isolated place into a world where he felt more accepted and empowered. Mario experienced a strong feeling of being alive in music whilst journeying towards his own death.

Surely it is because of the relationship between music and life that music therapy fits so readily in an environment where people face death, dying and all that this brings; that, when 'death is accorded its proper place – in the midst of life…' (Spence 1996), when a person is encouraged, enabled and celebrated as being whole, music can act as a very special agent. It is here, during musical improvisations in music therapy sessions, that life can be experienced in its rawest, truest sense.

Musicality

> ...musicality is not something one may have or not have, but something that...is constitutive of man. So defined, the concept cannot have a negative counterpart; to call a man unmusical would be meaningless, self-contradictory. Nobody is being singled out and set apart. Music is the concern of us all, not of a privileged elite... (Zuckerkand 1973, p.2)

Music therapy and the use of words within music therapy sessions is a current topic of active debate amongst music therapists. The experience of creating music is dramatically different from that of using words. Within the context of a music therapy session it is how we use words that is important. I have found over the years that my questions about the work have changed in a subtle, yet profound way. Instead of asking 'What is this music about for this person?' I find myself asking 'Why is it important for this person to experience themselves as being musical?' Here, I use the word 'musical' as being able to have an experience of oneself 'in music' – a time when one is not merely playing or singing along – but when one has reached a point when the music being improvised has a clear direction. This experience is not defined by skill and during these times, the therapist and patient will have an experience of flowing together in time, and both own a sensation of 'being carried along' by the music. If the musical experience is pre-eminent, the music therapist has a new and crucial responsibility. He should constantly remain open to the playing of the patient and be explicit in his own musical responses, should always pursue the development of his own improvisational skills, and should make a quest for the deepest understanding possible of musical experience. This is both an aesthetical (musical), and an ethical (therapeutic) imperative.

Patrick

I recall often that patients have been surprised by their ability to create music of an acceptable standard – surprised by their own 'musicality'. After completing an improvisation, Patrick, a thirty-year-old HIV positive recovering alcoholic, with no past experience of creating music, said:

> ...the sticks were in my hands and I was playing the xylophone. I had no idea what to do, but as if by magic they fell onto the instrument... I heard that you were playing the piano but what I played fitted in so perfectly. I was playing music, and it wasn't at all bad! ... The music had a life of it's own and we were being carried along by it...

Lindsay

> Sometimes, too, songs inspire us to look onwards and upwards, just for a moment they light the way, beckoning us, reminding us that we can keep faith; or that we can stay with the struggle – whatever it may be, taking risks, breaking new ground. Best of all perhaps, through songs we can touch again, however fleetingly, the essential truth that love changes everything. (Spence 1996, p.130)

Pre-composed music has played an important part during my work at Lighthouse – particularly songs. From time to time, patients would come to sessions wanting to perform a chosen pre-composed song. Even though during many of these performances it felt that the patient was pastiching a particular performer and maybe not truly being themselves, the effect was sometimes zealous and moving with a level of strength and self-acceptance being achieved.

Songs are often improvised too during therapy sessions. One example of this is the songs improvised together with a young woman. When I first met her, Lindsay was in her mid-twenties with a recent HIV positive diagnosis. She was referred to music therapy after a consultation appointment with the Lighthouse Homeopath during which she told him that she had been making up lyrics to songs in her head. She was perplexed by this as she had no experience of singing or practical music making in her past.

Lindsay arrived for her first music therapy session very depressed – her energy was low. When I suggested that we sang together, she declined saying that she could not sing. I played a note on the piano and asked if she could sing it, after a few moments she began to hum very quietly. I began to support her singing with sustained chords, gradually her sounds became more confident and words began to emerge. One of the questions that I find myself asking during a first improvisation with a patient is: 'What kind of musician does this person need me to be?' During this first session with Lindsay, I felt as if we were struggling to make contact – to find a musical language that we could experience together. At the conclusion of our first meeting she appeared surprised by what had happened. She said: 'It's as though a part of me I never knew existed has come to life'.

We agreed to make a contract to meet for six weekly sessions. When I saw her the following week there was a marked contrast in both her appearance and mood. She displayed more energy and began by singing confidently as she walked around the room.

What follows is a transcription of the lyrics to a song that she improvises. I accompany her from the piano and am struck by the simplicity of the accompaniment. The style of the music is something that I had not been used to – a simple chord progression I, Vi, IV, V and I with the occasional chord ii – the key is A Flat major and the tempo slow. Mostly her melody is based around the triadic formation of the chords that I use, but occasionally at high points in the harmonic direction she adds the leading note. Another point of interest comes at the moment when she sings the line '…and were gonna join.' Here, I begin to sing non-verbally with her:

> …If I dream about you the sky is full of stars,
> Oh…Mm… I'm floating higher, I'm going on.
> I'm floating higher, showering the stars,
> Floating around the rings of Mars.
> I'd like to be a big star,
> A twinkling little star in the sky.
> When the veil, black the veil, night comes down,
> Twinkling, twinkling, shining… (inaudible)
> And were gonna join (I sing non-verbally)
> A many splendid, happy, cosmic experience.
> When, on the ebb and flow of night and day,
> Oh how I pray.
> And I want to be you, so numb,
> I want to be a light and never glum,
> Oh that's immature! (Spoken)
> I can't realise, oh that this is life, that this is life,
> And it goes on, on and on and on…

During our post-improvisation discussion, we talked about the verbal content of the song. She told me that this was a song for her boyfriend. What is more interesting though, is the sense of harmonic and melodic structure that evolves within the improvisation, the new strength in the quality of her voice, and the reality that Lindsay experiences herself as being a singer. She was surprised by her own ability to create such songs, astonished by her own musicality. During the improvisations and also during the times when we listened back to the audio tapes together, she became more confident and her energy grew. Lindsay also visited a psychotherapist and we met on a number of occasions to discuss the work. Once, after sharing some of the audio-tapes with him, he said that there was no doubt in his mind that Lindsay's music therapy had a profound effect within her, helping her to come to terms with her diagnosis and to move on with her life. I continue to work with Lindsay from time to time on a short term basis. When she returns to music therapy it is always her own decision, and I am sure that it provides important experiences during periods when she is most vulnerable.

Boundaries

Boundaries are made in order to keep things safe. In ancient times, walls were built around towns and cities and along them people kept watch so that intruders and strangers were identified, any intent of harm being held at bay. In sport, boundaries are important so that both the players and spectators understand the rules of the game and fair play is maintained. In more recent years the word has taken on a number of meanings. Mostly they describe a line 'drawn around the outside' of certain experiences, events, and relationships. As Robert Frost (1930) says in his poem *Mending Wall:* 'Good fences make good neighbours' (p.47).

In therapy, the therapist and patient will agree at the outset on the terms of the therapeutic relationship; sessions will take place once or more a week, at a set time and within a set place. With such an agreement the therapeutic space is set up and boundaries are defined. What happens within the therapeutic space depends on the type of therapy that is being offered. Different boundaries are required around the different contexts within which different therapies take place.

In music therapy we rarely ask our patients to improvise music alone. We expect the patient to improvise music together with us and this defines the therapeutic relationship as being different from that of other therapies. For example, the basis of art therapy is that the patient produces an image and then, together with the therapist, statements and interpretations are made in order to make sense of that image which is assumed to be a manifestation of the patient's unconscious. Although the therapists' presence will often be an influence on both the patient and the image, it is unusual for them to be involved directly in its production. This allows the relationship to be less complicated and the boundaries to be more clear.

In music therapy, the involvement of the therapist as part of the improvisation means that the music is sounded together. The difference between improvising together and asking a patient to play alone highlights the uniqueness of the music therapeutic relationship. It gives the work a different foundation and most certainly an unparalleled outcome. There are a number of questions that arise out of this. 'Why is it important for the patient to play music together with us?' and 'What happens when we play music together?' When discussing music outside of therapy the same questions will emerge. 'Why do people play music together anyway?' and 'What happens when they do?' Attempts to understand these questions should remain at the heart of our work as music therapists.

The creation of music between people is a very intimate process and if we do not possess the deepest understanding of our art, emotional boundaries may become blurred. We should, therefore, be able to focus on how boundaries are identified and pinpointed within the music itself. Structure is an imperative component of music, and structure is defined by boundaries. Within musical structure we are in a world of rhythm, tonality, melody and harmony. Paul Nordoff, the pioneer music therapist, said in a BBC television documentary in 1976 that we are rhythmic and tonal beings, and rhythm and tone are the basic materials of music. This link between the components of music and the human condition provides an important basis for our work. It enables us to make a connection between the depths of our inner life and the breadth of the world outside of ourselves.

Musical components rest on a palette from which we are able to create and define the boundaries of our work. The boundaries available within music itself provide us with safety, security and our strength as therapists. Our confidence and competence as musicians is therefore of the utmost priority.

Adam

> When a person sings and cannot lift their voice, and another comes and sings with them, another who can lift their voice, then the first will be able to lift their voice too. That is the secret of the bond between spirit and spirit. (Gunzburg 1997, p.13)

I saw Adam once a week for four weeks before he died. He came to the music therapy room three times and the final session took place in his room on the residential unit. During the months before his death, Adam had grown increasingly forgetful and very confused. Sustaining a simple conversation was almost impossible and he displayed little awareness of where he was and who his closest friends were. Throughout his life he had enjoyed music immensely, and his strong relationship with it had been secured within a deep love for the opera. I agreed with his key nurse, that in order to work with Adam, a third person would be required to be present, as Adam was prone to unpredictable behaviour.

During the first session, the nurse himself sat in the room, with Adam's partner taking over this role during our final three meetings. The involvement of the third person was minimal – sitting quietly at the back of the therapy room allowing Adam and myself to improvise music together. What was surprising during the first three sessions, was the level of Adam's involvement. Although outside of the situation he was finding it difficult to sustain anything that required him to make contact with another person or persons, in music he was completely involved. He played a selection of drums for up to ten minutes, showing a high level of awareness of musical structure, of musical dynamics and changes in tempo. Once or twice, confidently and directly, he initiated a return to musical material that we had previously used. The person who was with us, whether it was Adam's partner or his key nurse, was surprised at his involvement, concentration, and level of commitment to the music. They were seeing a part of Adam which had ceased to be evident in other situations – the impulse to reach out to other people. When I arrived to see him for the fourth session I was told that since our last meeting he had become more and more withdrawn – to the point where he was no longer using speech at all and was finding it impossible to walk. Although both the key nurse and Adam's partner considered it important that we spent time together, it was now not possible to meet the therapy room. I would have to spend time with Adam on the residential unit and it proved difficult to find a period of time when this would be convenient. It was important that he was seen by the doctor and after that needed to be bathed. Initially, I arrived to see Adam at our appointed time just before lunch. We finally met around five o'clock in the evening.

The 'therapeutic space' that we had encountered during our previous sessions was no longer evident. The appointed time of our meeting, the space where his meeting was to take place, and the musical instruments were no longer an option. Adam was propped up in his bed, his partner sat on one side with myself on the other. I had taken no musical instruments and initially, we sat in silence together. Adam displayed no awareness that anyone was with him, staring straight ahead. After a short time, I began to sing non-verbally, my voice was soft, the tempo was slow, and I chose a simple four-phrase structure. Slowly Adam became involved. Firstly he directed his gaze towards me and then, with an enormous amount of effort began to sing. He sang intermittently to begin with, mostly at the end of phrases. Gradually it became more sustained and I felt that he was motivated by the simplicity of the musical structure. Spontaneously, his partner began to sing with us, and for a time the three of us were together in music; it was an intensely emotional experience.

Much later, after the funeral, I spoke to his partner. He believed that the singing had been an important experience for both of them, as he felt it was the last time they had truly made a connection with each other.

Within an environment such as Lighthouse, boundaries need to be flexible. If they are not, their rigidity can damage if not halt, the therapeutic process. I have no doubt that with Adam, our experience within the final session was therapeutically valid and that we were held, firstly within the safety of the boundaries created in the music itself, and secondly within the structural and philosophical boundaries of a steadfast institution.

Endings

> An HIV diagnosis presses…buttons, and asks…questions: Why are we here? What will happen when I die? Is there a God?…But most of all it presses the button of fear. Will death be endless night? Endless pain? Or perhaps worse than that: Endless nothing? (Woodward 1991, p.57)

Before working at Lighthouse, the majority of my experience as a music therapist had been in child, adolescent and adult mental health, and physical and mental disability. Prior to the music therapy training, I had worked as a counsellor and during the early years as a therapist had struggled to combine the two disciplines. In comparison to working in mental health, I found the musical improvisations I experienced at Lighthouse had a directness and clarity that I had not witnessed before; I was struck by a new concept of time. When patients came for music therapy sessions, there appeared to be less trepidation and a more concrete knowing. It was as if these people (the majority of whom had no experience of creating music and certainly no experience of what music therapy might be), knew what they wanted from it more clearly and more directly than I had encountered before. Whereas in the past, I had been used to long periods of exploration, apparent confusion and some sense of struggle with patients, at Lighthouse I felt that they played mostly for the moment with a high level of energy, passion and commitment.

Adrian

Adrian was a case in point. In his mid-thirties, he had been a stalwart user of the organisation since its earliest days and had some previous experiences of music therapy. He had sat on numerous committees, worked as a volunteer, and had stood up for the principles of the institution during difficult and demanding times. He was one of the many gay, HIV positive men who had been empowered – inspired even – by the Lighthouse philosophy; belonging to this community had given him hope and had changed his life.

I was in my first weeks of work with those living with HIV/AIDS when Adrian arrived for his initial music therapy session. My impressions were of a man who was forthright and determined. As I began to explain to him what music therapy could be, a practice that I have long since revised, he began arranging the percussion instruments around himself in a large cluster. I continued to talk, but appearing not to listen, he picked up a pair of drum sticks and, cutting across my monologue, began to play the instruments with an enormous amount of vigour. I rushed to the piano and began to improvise with him. I shall never forget this first time of hearing him play the percussion instruments. It was loud and constant, hardly letting up for a moment, and was driven by an immense energy. Repetition of any kind was infrequent and I found it difficult to musically grasp hold of anything that he played. During our early meetings together these improvisations were astronomic, lasting for the entire fifty to sixty minute sessions. It was all I could do to reflect back the strength of his playing from the piano. I remember being surprised by the silence at the end of each session. Any verbal response from Adrian would be monosyllabic and he would leave the room without discussion of the musical improvisations.

I can recall the frustration I felt when improvising with him. I tried hard to make sense of it musically, attempting to mould it into something more concrete and meaningful in the hope that it would give Adrian a sense of being supported and held. From time to time, whether playing the piano or the percussion instruments with him, I would halt completely. There would be no response from Adrian, and he would continue playing with the same, ongoing frenzy of sound.

A key point came during the third month of working together. Out of my frustration of improvising with him, I began to question the validity of such work. Here he was having a cathartic experience, no doubt, but with seemingly no moments of musical connection with myself. In my opinion, music therapy was about a relationship. When truly relating in music therapy there should be some periods of mutual recognition of the interpersonal moments of musical connection. During the eleventh session, after about twenty minutes of such percussion playing, Adrian moved to the marimba. His playing was loud and lacked any sense of tonality or structure. For a time I played the piano with him trying desperately to work out what he meant (musically) by it. Out of my frustration I stood up and, taking a beater hit the marimba, directly cutting across his playing. He stopped:

Is that a therapeutic technique? he exclaimed. Silence.

Are you upset because I invaded your space? I asked. Silence.

No, he answered, only because what you did had nothing to do with what I was playing! (Adrian, Session 11, March 1993)

Of course, depending on how we view music therapy, there are a number of ways to perceive the above incident. One might say that what I did was to offer a classic interpretation or intervention. If we listen with respect to what he says though, we hear that he is responding to an insensitive musical reaction on my part, giving him the message that what he was doing was not acceptable.

This event had a profound effect on me as a music therapist. Here, I am talking of things that are commonly described as musical and extra-musical. There is an enormous difference between making an informed musical intervention during therapeutic improvisation, offering changes in tempo, dynamic, tonal centre, metre etc. with the intention of presenting new musical experiences and challenges to the patient, and crude, physical, extra-musical gestures which at best will have little effect, or at worst, tactlessly destroy the creative endeavour and display a lack of respect towards the patient.

Adrian's verbal response, and how I reacted to it, had an effect on our work together – it was a defining moment. He told me that for many years he had listened to and admired the compositions of musicians such as Cornelius Cardew and Eddie Prevost. These were the musicians from which he was drawing inspiration for our improvisations together. The understanding of Adrian's previous relationship with music was an important one. Instead of making an interpretation that the disordered percussion playing reflected the quality of his inner life, I could now see that here was a person making a conscious musical choice. Of course this conscious musical choice doesn't occur with every patient, but as I discovered, we would do well as music therapists to consider the music of our patients in such a way. We should bear in mind that all of our patients come to us with their own unique relationship to music, and this can have an effect on the music created during therapy sessions.

As we continued working together, Adrian's playing of the percussion instruments did not change, it was present during most of the times we met over a period of two and a half years. What did alter was my perception of this playing, enabling us to meet within it in a more dynamic and respectful way. This change, which without doubt came from an alteration of how we both listened to each other within music, also helped us to move forward into other worlds of musical improvisation. Timing – the point when a change in the music would occur – and waiting for that point became the central cores of our work.

Over our time together, Adrian and I explored many different styles and flavours of music. He demanded from me a flexibility in musical language that was sometimes frightening but always inspiring. It was as if we were truly on a journey together flying through the air, not knowing where we would land or what our next musical experience would be.

Endings play a large part, not only in music therapy sessions, but also within the organisation of Lighthouse as a whole. If someone has died during the day, a candle will be lit in their memory and placed on the reception desk – a constant reminder of our mortality. Also a memorial book is available, set in a quiet space for loved ones, friends, patients, staff and visitors to record thoughts or personal messages to those who have died.

The end of a therapeutic relationship can come in a number of ways. At Lighthouse, they have rarely been planned. I remember during my early work when deaths were more frequent, needing personally to regard every session as an entity in itself. Long term therapeutic aims and goals were sometimes pointless and I even tried not to plan the following weeks sessions with some patients. Often there would be no opportunity to say 'good-bye' or to bring the work to an end in any formal way – this now happens to a lesser extent. Regularly I would be asked to provide music at a patient's funeral, sometimes playing audio recordings of improvisations which had been created during music therapy sessions as part of the ritual if this had been their wish. I began to find that this could be a peremptory way of saying 'good-bye' and bringing the music therapeutic relationship to an end.

Adrian and I worked together for two and a half years before he died – the length of time being unusual in comparison with most patients who were more ill when I had my first contact with them. During our work, Adrian had been very ill on a number of occasions, but he had always pulled through. He was a long term survivor of the virus.

Our final session together could not have been known as such by either of us. Adrian had been in good health, but during the six days after what was to be our last music therapy session together, the virus entered his brain and he died suddenly. When I heard of his death I was shocked and somewhat confused. I felt that our work had not finished and there was more to be done. I decided to listen to the tape of our last session in the hope that it might provide some explanation. As I listened I was not struck by anything until the final one and a half minutes. During these final one and a half minutes, Adrian plays the piano and I play the percussion instruments. Initially I sense an unease in the both our playing; it was a combination to which we were unused. Suddenly the quality of Adrian's sound changes – the quality of his touch on the keys – and he begins to repeat three notes over and over. He starts with his right hand on F sharp (above middle C), moving up a fifth to C sharp, and then down an augmented fourth to G natural. The dynamic is soft, the tempo is slow, and the notes are placed with cut-glass precision. Throughout I am playing an almost inaudible bass drum roll. Finally Adrian brings in his left hand with sustained, descending clusters ending in the utmost bass register of the piano. The sound eventually dies away and we sit quietly together.

Here I am reminded of where I began. Musical improvisation defies verbal interpretation. There is something very significant about the final moments of our musical relationship. Repetition of any kind had been completely alien to our music making, and here Adrian was not only repeating a musical idea but doing so in a simple and deliberate way. Also at the end of improvisations it had become customary for Adrian to physically move from where he was almost instantly and to walk around the room. After this final improvisation we sat together for a longer period of time. Whenever I have played this audio tape to people the reaction to it has always been profound. Even taking into account that in retrospect, it is always easy to hear what we want to, and as a therapist I was looking to make sense of the ending to a therapeutic journey, it is difficult to say why it is so effective – it defies definition. On some level the music does truly speak for itself.

> I still have my idealism and my hopes about the way I would like the world to be. Perhaps people will never live together in a community, co-operatively and in harmony…Perhaps a real and true response to AIDS

can help to create a better world, a truly supportive, loving community where people can be creative together. (Woodward 1991, p.52)

Coda

Lighthouse has been described as a community many times over the years. Within a true community each person is valued and respected for who they are and a sense of balance between people is constantly striven for. The act of creating music, as so clearly put by Mario during our work together, can create a feeling of being in balance – both a feeling of balance between therapist and client and also a feeling of balance within oneself. He talks convincingly of an intensified experience of life whilst journeying towards his own death, not a denial of death but an acceptance of it as being central to human existence – 'I never felt so alive!' When listening to the words and improvisations of such patients during and after music therapy sessions, I realise that from out of the isolation of an HIV positive diagnosis, the improvisation of music can assist in moving beyond denial and offer glimmers of hope, an installation of well-being, a fostering of courage in the face of adversity and a new and animated understanding of both life and death.

The creation of music can never be an isolated act, even when playing music alone we are relating to the world around us – it is the most social of the arts. Therefore the experience of making music should be paramount to human existence. It is from out of the contact we have with other people that we can begin to value who and what we are and glimpse the potential of who and what we can be. Music offers a direct and uncomplicated medium for being close together, a medium within which participants can be respected, revered and even celebrated. Thomas Mann defines music as a 'manifestation of the highest energy not as idea, rather in its actuality...' (1949, p.78). In making a direct connection between music and God, he places it alongside some of the greatest mysteries of human existence. In bringing energy into being, making it audible, acceptable and real, we embrace the central and most important strength of music therapy.

I call your attention to the fact that this is almost the definition of God. Imitatio Dei – I am surprised that is not forbidden... I do not like to call it beautiful, the word beauty has always been offensive to me...and people feel wanton and corrupt when they say it. But it is good, good in the extreme, it could not be better...it ought not be better. (Mann 1949, pp. 78–79)

London Lighthouse not only offers a convincing philosophy for the world of HIV/AIDS, but a philosophy for life.

CHAPTER 9

Music Therapy with HIV Positive and AIDS Patients

Lutz Neugebauer

Music therapy was swiftly absorbed into the fields of neurology, psychiatry, psychosomatics and inner medicine following the work initiated by Paul Nordoff and Clive Robbins (1977). In the general hospital at Herdecke, music therapy became an integrated element in the treatment of patients with various medical complaints (Aldridge 1989; Aldridge and Verney 1988; Gustorff 1990, 1992a, 1992b, 1996; Lichtenberger 1993; Neugebauer 1993, 1995; Schnürer *et al.* 1995).

Seeing illness as not just a physical condition, taking into account the change in the human self-regulatory capacity both physically and psychologically, clarifies the way art therapies can be understood. Patients are able to find new ways of returning to being active and creative through their artistic endeavours. The basis of my approach to music therapy is the joint improvisation of patient and therapist. Musical communication reunites them both as parts of a whole, as in a chamber music performance where different voices contribute to a complete sound. By careful listening to each other, what is being heard can be put back actively into the music. Further development is dependent on the personal capabilities of both participants. There is a synchronised process of sensory impression, feeling, intent and expression between patient and therapist (Neugebauer 1998).

The individual character of each improvisation expresses the patient's condition and state of health. Since the network of relationships has been developed within the music, it is possible to describe all events in musical terms. These descriptions supersede the measurable, since they are of a qualitative nature, but they can nevertheless be objectified by means of tape-recorded documentation. The patient's music-making reveals both limitations and possibilities, and it is up to the therapist to hear, discern, discover, and encourage. Music therapy gives a patient the opportunity of objectively experiencing his own state of health, of which he is otherwise only aware of on an introspective and subjective level of perception, and at whose mercy he finds himself because of his illness. In addition, this experience opens up in him the possibility of bringing about active change, that is, of grasping and developing musical opportunities for change. As a result there is active participation in the healing process. The patient becomes active instead of merely being given treatment.

This consideration was one of the main reasons for the inclusion of music therapy in the treatment of people whose main problem was the weakening or breakdown of their immune system from a medical point of view, but whose individual personal problems extended far beyond this.

When we come into contact with AIDS patients, or those that are immunologically challenged, we are meeting people whose lives are overshadowed by death. In contrast to other diseases, for instance cancer, the victims can very often give a precise description of when, where, and why they contracted their illness. This gives rise to the question of 'atonement' or paying the price for ones way of life that some patients ask. Here we see how necessary an impartial, fearless discourse is for all concerned, so that normal contacts with mutual respect can become possible.

For the individual patient, diagnosed as HIV positive, this diagnosis is a turning-point in his life. Patients are often forced into a dilemma of whether to go for treatment or to keep their diagnosis a secret, in order to avoid dreaded consequences. AIDS is a feared disease, not least as a result of the extensive information campaigns, and patients find themselves at a cross-roads. The diagnosis transforms social and intimate relationships radically, not just reactively, but sometimes also at the patients instigation. Planning the future would seem to have very limited possibilities, maybe not short term, but certainly with the prospect of repeated, often prolonged hospital stays. The unequivocal prognoses of debilitating physical handicaps and psychiatric disturbances are bound to disrupt any forward-looking activities, especially in the acute phases in which we meet the patients.

Because the future for the immune-challenged appears to be radically curtailed, therapies that involve creative processes and incorporate patients potentials seem to be most appropriate in promoting hope. This is particularly true taken that art therapies are experience-related, not being dependant on a verbal approach, and the mental conflicts already besetting the patient, and not focusing on physical disablement or changes in laboratory findings, which are literally a matter of life and death for the patient. The involvement of non-verbal art therapies is a special way of caring for the patient not just on a medical nursing level, but also by weaving in a unique form of psychological and spiritual care (Aldridge 1993).

First experiences

Nearly all patients entering hospital after initial out-patient consultations willingly and unreservedly accept the offer of music therapy. Whether the patient is wheeled in his bed to the music therapy room or is able to get there by himself, the aim is always to improvise music together. A dialogue is developed in the literal sense, as an 'exchange of ideas' (Neugebauer 1998). The ensuing music depends entirely on the patient's individual possibilities, using various instruments. After initial shyness patients often experience immediate pleasure which is reflected in their music-making.

Descriptions of music are by definition difficult; their abstract nature eludes verbal expression. However, we have to try as therapists to describe what we do for others that may be interested. The music-making of two patients is described below. It is not my intent to generalise about all immunologically challenged patients that are HIV positive from these case studies, simply to reflect through two examples how music therapy can help. Each patient comes to me as an individual and we make music together, the person takes the foreground and the disease assumes a background role. The person is more important than the disease, or perhaps we might say 'humans before viruses'.

The following work is based on creative improvised music therapy that assumes an active part in the music making by the patient. No matter how physically challenged a person may be, it is possible to move some part of the body such that an instrument can be struck (Ansdell 1995). In this approach the therapist is predominantly playing the piano.

Example one

Mr K starts to play with a single drumstick, standing in front of a drum and cymbal. I join in at the piano later, taking up dominant elements of his playing. On the drum he plays a one-bar rhythmical motive, which he repeats several times unchanged. The sound is dull, edgy, stodgy, and dynamically monotonous. When I accompany him on the piano from the fourth bar on, with a bass motive taking up the main rhythmic impulses, he immediately loses the form, which we are however able to regain in a Spanish-style of music. However Mr K needs a lot of musical assistance to keep up continuous playing. Metrically unstructured music, which might be considered as an alternative, makes him so insecure that he stops playing each time he is confronted with it.

Since he is sure that his difficulties are caused by technical problems using the drumstick, for the next improvisation he chooses bongos. He plays these with both hands. His playing is irregular and sounds clumsy. It is full of changing accents and continuous tempo variations. The change between left and right hands is uncoordinated and he gets faster. But, when I accompany him – note for note with runs and arpeggios, in unison an octave apart in romantic style – there is initial musical contact. This is the contact he seems to have been searching for. He enjoys playing the accelerating runs until they get too fast for him. He stops and starts all over again. His repeated loss of control over the tempo is incorporated into a rubato improvisation, again in a romantic style, which is repeated in later sessions.

In the fourth session a new element is introduced when Mr K superimposes his own tempi and phrasing on the romantic style, taking the initiative to use the cymbal for accents, finding clear beginnings, endings and musical climaxes. His manual co-ordination is so good that he can play according to an anticipatory musical plan of action.

Mr K was discharged from the hospital after four weeks treatment, in a considerably improved state of health.

Example two

Mr B is too weak to come to the music therapy room by himself, so I fetch him at his express wish, wheeling him in his hospital bed to the therapy room. On the way there he hands me the score of a choral motet he would like me to play and sing for him. In the therapy room he tries many times to sing fragments of it but has to break off because of breathing difficulties. However, he gesticulates for me to carry on. After the first part of the piece he tells me tearfully that he is no longer even able to do things he is familiar with, so I will have to sing for him instead.

I care for Mr B for seven weeks by making music with him twice weekly in the therapy room for as long as his deteriorating condition allows, then in his hospital room. Mr B's relationships with the hospital staff are strained but during the music therapy sessions he becomes calm and approachable. One session, I take a selection of music to him. Without even looking at my music he asks me to sing to him the Bach chorale 'Jesus, my joy', which I happen to have brought with me. I accompany my own singing on the cembalo. He holds a copy of the chorale in his weakened hands and follows the words of the first two verses:

> Jesus my joy,
> my hearts pasture,
> Jesus my treasure.
> Ah, how long, how long
> Has the heart been afraid and longing for you.
> Lamb of God, my Lord,
> Nothing on earth shall be better loved than you.
> In your protection I am safe from the onslaughts
> of all enemies.
> Let Satan curse,
> let the world tremble,
> Jesus is with me.
> When there is thunder and lightning,
> When sin and hell frighten,
> Jesus will protect me.

With great exertion he joins in the singing of the third verse:

> Defy the aged dragon,
> defy deaths revenge,
> defy fear.
> Let the world rage and fall,
> I will stand here and sing
> in your safe haven....

at which point he says firmly: 'That's enough, thank you.'

Next day Mr B dies.

Although these two examples are very different, they do show similar 'musical traits'. Both patients have seemingly lost their personal concept of continuous time, or at least their ability to express it externally. Music offered unique opportunities to both: for one the chance to be actively creative in sickness, for the other the experience of confronting death and dying in a way not accessible to him at any other level. Both descriptions show that music can open up opportunities for communication and relationships beyond the spoken word.

Therapists and patients play together as music-making peers. Structures involving leading and following, and synchronised complementary playing, can make joint music-making possible.

Example three

Music therapy started for Mr W during his first stay in hospital and was continued throughout all ensuing stays. In the first phase of music therapy treatment, Mr W had two sessions per week. This arrangement continued during later stays, although he was not always able to attend both sessions, depending on his state of health.

From the earliest sessions, which Mr W attends readily, musical idiosyncrasies are apparent and develop into an integral and operative part of his entire music therapy treatment. Mr W's playing on melodic percussion shows great sensitivity, which he expresses through delicate playing during quieter passages. His playing floats without a recognisable outer structure and the therapist accompanies him with open, atonal and unbound music resulting in a spontaneous duet.

Diametrically opposite to this sensitive side of his playing, we have his musical interpretation on percussive instruments such as the drum and cymbals, which is predominantly loud and hard. He plays single beats, which appear very stable in sequence, but lack tempo in a musical sense being seemingly unrelated to each other. In volume or tempo changes his playing becomes even harder. Continuous progress is almost impossible and development is step-by-step.

In both kinds of playing it is apparent that he doesn't seem able to dictate what happens in the music. Once established, musical routines could go on for ever if they didn't lead to physical exhaustion and have to be broken off. There is hardly any evidence of the therapist's improvisations influencing changes or formal structures, which is astonishing considering the apparent sensitivity I hear in the playing.

During the first group of sessions it becomes increasingly clear that Mr W is aware of these discrepancies. For this reason, one of the elements he works on musically in all the sessions is form-finding and this leads to the structure of transitions and conclusions. With the help of musical suggestions contributed by me, he discovers in himself an increasing ability to include musically these elements of transition.

He always enjoys the music therapy sessions even though he is physically and mentally exhausted afterwards. He describes how he is hearing his own music and how he meets himself in this music. But over and beyond this meeting, he can see the possibilities of actively intervening in what confronts him. After the first session he says that for this reason of active intervention, music therapy is more important to him than the various kinds of psychotherapy he has experienced.

The musical aspects also dominate the second block of music therapy treatment sessions four months later. More evidently than in the earlier sessions, Mr W finds endings and conclusions with the help of the improvised music. He always manages to actively intervene when his own music is taken up, and the dominant elements of it emphasised, without having to interrupt the musical flow.

At the beginning of the third treatment block, six months later, the dominant musical impression comprises, once more, unformed, disintegrated playing. But, Mr W very quickly reproduces the musical possibilities achieved during his previous hospitalisation. For the first time there are phases of mutually imitative dialogue and resting periods in his playing. These pauses are lengthened by means of musical elements introduced by me that result for the first time in deliberate conclusions and conscious new beginnings. After a certain amount of adjustment, Mr W is also able to compose rondo forms (a-b-a-c-a-d-a-e-a). Recognition and repetition, beyond the purely mechanical level, are the distinguishing features of this improvisation phase.

This time Mr W leaves the hospital asking how he can apply his ability in music and art therapy to take the initiative and act independently in the rest of his life.

During his next hospitalisation period he again carries on where he left off at the previous music therapy sessions, but his fluctuating physical condition make continuous work impossible. The treatment even has to be broken off at times because Mr W refuses to let me make music for him in his room.

The first session after a long period of being bedridden, six months later, takes up where the previous ones left off. He is obviously very weak. He is able to play flexibly, yet can influence his own playing and appears self-confident in the musical dialogue. At this point he decides, in consultation with all his carers in the team, to continue music therapy as his sole therapy form. Up to his discharge he has two sessions weekly. He is autonomous within the therapy and enjoys its recreational aspects.

In the last hospitalisation period, he also has music therapy. This time he calls me for the first time for an appointment of his own volition. He is also able to carry on where he left off after his last hospitalisation. Although he sees his whole life situation as depressingly sad, during music therapy he takes great pleasure in his confidence in playing and enjoys being accompanied in varying styles (from oriental music to clog-dancing). Not only can he join in with varying moods and styles but he can also intentionally instigate them. In lively music, he can change directions after following for a short time, and in this way he plays an indispensable and vital role as an equal in the musical whole. He recognises and savours situations in which the music attains the level of social communication and is always sorry when the therapy sessions come to an end. I always decide when to end the sessions and Mr W only becomes aware how strenuous the work is physically and emotionally when we leave the therapy room.

We have arranged to continue the music therapy during future periods of hospitalisation.

Further thoughts

Many patients develop distinctly neurological symptoms because of their immunological breakdown. Music therapy can here offer possibilities similar to those of the early creative music therapy work (Nordoff and Robbins 1977). For instance, patients who lose the ability to speak, live in a social isolation similar to that of the children for whom music therapy was originally evolved. Music therapy encourages an articulation that lies beyond the use of words.

Music therapy has a significant role to play in the treatment of HIV positive patients. Not only does music therapy offer an existential form of therapy that accepts the person as he or she is, and an opportunity to define him or herself as he or she wishes to be, it is primarily concerned with aesthetic issues of form and existential notions of potential rather than concepts of pathology. That the person is infected with a virus recalcitrant to medical initiatives, is given and inarguable. What the person will become and how a personal future is defined, a future which is admittedly restricted and often tragically curtailed, are matters for joint therapeutic endeavour between therapist and patient and are not accessible to a normative medical science (Aldridge 1996).

Creative music therapy opens up a unique possibility to take an initiative in coping with disease, or to find a level to cope with near death. Rather than the patient living in the realm of pathology alone, they are encouraged to find the realm of their own creative being.

If the progress of this disease, AIDS, is an increasing personal isolation then the therapeutic relationship is an important one for maintaining interpersonal contact. A contact which is morally non-judgmental, where the ground of that contact is aesthetic and expressive, not scientific and repressive. Patients are allowed to be as they are, to realise themselves in a musical context that allows them to reach their potential.

CHAPTER 10

The Implications of Melodic Expression for Music Therapy with a Breast Cancer Patient

Gudrun Aldridge

This chapter deals with the question of what contribution music therapy can make to the treatment of a breast cancer patient after she has been treated for the removal of a breast. In particular, the musical aspect of melody will be discussed in the role it plays for facilitating expression.

We know from the literature that it is important for breast cancer patients to be able to express themselves. We also know that melody in our modern culture is an important form of expression. If expression is important for breast cancer patients, and melody is an important form of musical expression, then it makes sense to develop the melodic playing of patients in music therapy.

In the following chapter, I offer a brief view of the meaning of cancer in our Western society putting an emphasis on the salient features of the appropriate literature to gain a broader perspective of the complexity of the disease. A case study demonstrates the possibilities that melodic improvisation brings, exemplifying the melodic development in the therapy as we improvise together, and illustrates the relevant nuances of the patient's emotional expressivity. The work described here is taken from when I was working as a music therapist at the oncological ward of a general hospital that includes anthroposophical medicine alongside conventional medical treatment in the treatment program.

The disease in context

Breast cancer is the second leading cause of cancer incidence and mortality for women. Out of approximately 200 different kinds of cancerous diseases, breast cancer among women is the most widespread and increasing in incidence. Cancer is regarded not only as an illness but also as a malicious, invincible enemy that can threaten ones own life and prospects of promotion in working life (Sontag 1993). The experience of breast cancer in our society, in which the breast of the woman is a part of the cultural code for femininity and sexuality, is a very deep one and can cause psychic trauma (Wear 1993). In facing a potentially fatal disease, a woman is terrified to loose a precious part of her body that is deeply embedded in her sexuality and femininity.

Of the varying events that are feared most are mutilation or amputation of one part of the body, the pain attached to that amputation, the uncertainty about the success of treatment, the possibility of the diseases recurrence, a deterioration of the condition, and death. To be faced with these events and possibilities causes deep and significant feelings 'that cannot be medicalised into neat stage theories or normalised by upbeat assurances' (Wear 1993, p.82).

At a time of increasing uncertainty, questions about guilt and ones own abnormal behaviour occur. Things one is afraid of, or which are felt as an insult or repulsion, may easily be identified with the disease. Susan Sontag (1993) sees cancer as being used by society as a metaphor for moralising upon things that are seen as wrong. Similarly, Wilkinson sees it as no coincidence that this disease is often viewed within a moral context (Wilkinson and Kitzinger 1993), as we saw in the previous two chapters. A feature that has always been present in society is the attempt to combine the individual's point of view with a moral secular view that reflects upon the existence of good and bad people. In transferring upon this moral perspective to the body and health concerns, opinions are often expressed that describe 'unharmonious' individuals as susceptible to diseases. In this way the attribution of illness becomes a kind of moral judgement about the degree of control an individual has over her life.

The psychological effect of life threatening diseases, like cancer, has been intensively examined in different psycho-oncological research studies with various emphases; such as psychological, psychosocial or coping research (Berti, Hoffmann and Mbus 1993; Carter 1993; Carter and Carter 1993; Carter, Carter and Prosen 1992; Geyer 1993; Hürny et al. 1993; Nelson et al.

1994; Rawnsley 1994; Shapiro *et al.* 1994; Stanton and Snider 1993, Wong and Bramwell 1992).

The diagnosis of cancer can precipitate a state of profound anxiety that is associated with sensitivity, vulnerability, hopelessness, thoughts about death and uncertainty about the future (Wong and Bramwell 1992). An aim of the previously mentioned research has been to establish valid psychodynamic and psychosocial effective indicators that can give information about the course of the disease.

There is an increasing assumption that points to a correlation between mental events and the dissemination and progressive development of cancer. As Spiegel's (1991) study shows, many other research studies have in fact demonstrated that suppression of, and the inability to express, anger is in some ways associated with the appearance of cancer. Spiegel does not argue that cancer can be caused by this inability to express anger. Nonetheless, there are indicators in the literature suggesting that survival and disease progression can be influenced by psychosocial interventions. Spiegel himself examined the effect of a psychosocial intervention on mood and pain, and discovered a positive effect on these variables. He found that there was not only reduced mood disturbance and less pain, but less phobic and better coping responses as well. For him the value and advantage of psychosocial intervention is the fundamental improvement of the woman's quality of life.

Carter (1994) too points out the importance of a wider social context. In her article she presents an example case of the problematic work re-entry experience for a breast cancer survivor. She concludes that social stigma and discrimination lead to isolation, and both contribute to a negative view of the situation many working women are confronted with. The negative experience of going back to work may cause a problem of reconstructing a positive sense of self. Carter discusses the possibilities that facilitate a return to work and suggests recommendations for the further development of work re-entry programs.

Subjective well-being is a major aspect of quality of life that is influenced to a great extent by the complex process of coping with the disease and its treatment (Hürny *et al.* 1993). When we are faced with unusual, extreme demands, like serious life events or life-threatening diseases, the question of coping with the life-threatening problem comes to the fore. Within the framework of coping research, coping strategies, that are closely connected with the disease, become an increasing topic of research. Defence mechanisms are not only seen as an intrapsychic event, but also in connection with the social context of a burdening life situation (Berti, Hoffmann and Möbus 1993).

A cancer diagnosis is particularly stressful (Stanton and Snider 1993). It requires that women make potentially life-altering decisions regarding treatment rapidly. Because of this urgency, avoidant coping may impede effective cognitive processing and problem solving activities that are directed towards those decisions. Stanton suggests that care providers should encourage social support and points to directions for research on supportive interventions with cancer patients.

Creative music therapy appears to be a particularly pertinent form of adjuvant therapy that encourages supportive relationships and offers the woman a chance to participate actively in her own treatment.

The implications of psychosocial research for music therapy practice

What we can take from the literature about breast cancer is the fact that psychological and social factors are important aspects and have a crucial influence on the post-operative phase. The best possible medical treatment is a radical one (amputation, radiation/chemotherapy), and is not sufficient to provide the patients with the most possible healing chances. Medical treatment alone cannot be content with surgery and radiation but has to include, and offer, other psychosocial interventions that enable women to find a way how to handle their disease, and the consequences of medical intervention. Of these interventions, an emphasis can be made on enabling women to find their own perspectives on the disease and encourage a new integration in their own biography. The increasing number of long term studies clarifies the seriousness of this aspect and shows how the emphasis of these research studies has shifted to include the view of the persons effected. From this personal individualised point of view it is hoped to give better and more effective recommendations for supportive after-care.

Creative music therapy could be a valuable contribution to meet the patient's different needs. With its individual approach, it meets the results of Nelson and colleagues (Nelson et al. 1994), who demonstrate that patients with very different adjustment profiles, and less emotional distress, profit remarkably from individually tailored psychosocial interventions.

When confronted with the diagnosis of cancer, and its medical follow-up, women experience and suffer a number of events that may also bring about serious changes. Fundamental questions emerge about how to deal with the body after amputation; how to deal with the emotional suffering that ensues; how to cope with the image that remains of an altered body; and how to handle the consequent social and professional problems (reorganising the life at home within the family, communicating with family, friends and acquaintances, dealing with possible financial difficulties). Furthermore, there is a problem of how to deal with the distance other people place between themselves and the sufferer, and the distance the sufferer may feel towards her own body. By neglecting personal needs (Carter 1994), feelings of isolation and distance from ones own body and illness can emerge. In becoming aware of her own intrinsic feelings during the actual musical playing, music therapy provides possibilities to promote an intimacy for the woman with her own body, and create an artistic dialogue to reinforce and activate interpersonal communication.

Music therapy may also provide the opportunity to become active creatively, to develop new orientation and direction in the patients life (Aldridge, Brandt and Wohler 1990) Heyde and v. Langsdorff (1983) also propose that by using a therapy program that is active and perceptive at the same time, music therapy helps to experience ones own undreamt-of capabilities and offers the chance to develop new strength.

Anxiety and *depression* are often cited as the predominant affective pattern in facing cancer. Patients are forced by their disease to know how to deal with their own emotional reactions. Some may succeed better than others, depending upon their nature. Music, while having everything to do with emotion, has nothing to do with the labels 'anxiety', 'depression' or 'aggression'. Music therapy has the effect of offering clients space and possibilities to express themselves directly out of their difficult situation, without normative expectations and without the fear of judgement of doing everything wrong (Sontag 1993). It is presumed here that therapists are basing their reactions on acceptance, as we have seen in the two previous chapters, and not on moral judgements.

In having the ability to play as one feels in a creative way, there is a chance for women to achieve a sense of a new identity. To perform musically as an active manifestation of self, may itself contribute to mood improvement and reduce negative feelings like despair, depression, loneliness and anxiety. David Aldridge (1996) suggests that in music therapy patients can find their own way of expression that is creative and not limited by an illness. To start out from this way of looking, one could expect to find indicators that in spite of a deterioration of the physical parameters, point to an improvement of life quality. This would be of special value for breast cancer patients.

In this context, an interesting insight is given by Aldridge's phenomenological comparison between the organisation of music and the self that sees a correlation between music form and biological form. In proposing a phenomenological understanding that is isomorphic with the medium of music itself, he stresses the qualitative and non-verbal features of a holistic consciousness that is participatory and appears in the very phenomenon of music as performed. He assumes that in hearing music the phenomenon becomes, as direct experience, its own explanation. People can be understood as they come into the world as music, e.g. composed as physiological and psychological 'whole' beings. In using a musical metaphor it is possible for him to look at human identities as 'symphonic' that are continuously composed in the moment as opposed to a 'mechanic' view that regards the physical body as a being that has to be repaired. With this Aldridge reveals concrete possibilities for a new way of looking at the use of creative music therapy, where 'personality types' are not limitations but themes in a repertoire of being. He suggests that we consider the premise 'I perform, therefore I am', in contrast to the Cartesian idea of, 'I think, therefore I am'.

The possibility of self-awareness and self-experience, which the literature suggests is problematic for breast cancer patients, can be achieved through playing music. The use of creative music therapy allows women to become aware of the ground of their being, to reach their own deep world of expression and allow their identity to be revealed. An exploration of such depths could lead to the release of some emotions, especially those of anxiety and anger, and the promotion of others, such as hope and joy. In experiencing ones entire self a woman is not only 'playing' her physical weakness and affliction but expressing her individual potential in the moment. Women may experience themselves in improvised musical playing not only as physically restricted by infirmity, but as a transcended being herself realised in the music (Aldridge 1996). This phenomenological approach allows therapists to experience patients with their potential for health and well-being and therefore has a vital and vitalising effect in the therapeutic process.

The music therapeutic process, with its various demands and changes is a joint effort. The function of the music therapist, as the following examples show, is that she is pointing the way for new modes of expression and in the context of the musical relationship, allowing a new identity to emerge. Within a context of musical communication, flexibility of expression may be encouraged within a supportive musical form. Music therapy offers a powerful tool for promoting communication in terms of personal and interpersonal integration. This would counteract the aspect of isolation that is mentioned in the literature. By the use of creative dialogues, interpersonal contact is maintained, and patient's experience that they are not estranged within themselves, or estranged from others.

Looking from a holistic perspective, improvised music therapy appears to meet the needs of women during various stages of the illness. Music therapy, as a receptive and an active intervention, can bring physical relief (reduce fatigue, powerlessness, and help to distract from pain); influence emotional stressors positively, transforming feelings from negative to positive, enhance mood and reduce suffering; promote an awareness of intimacy with the body; encourage a new personal orientation and stimulate a new personal direction; encourage a creative musical dialogue by enhancing the modes of expression, and promoting flexibility of expressive response, personally and in relationships; and reduce social difficulties by encouraging interpersonal contact and reducing isolation (Aldridge 1996).

Music therapy then, with its possibilities of intervention, support, affirmation, distraction, confrontation and communication, represents a meaningful form of therapy adjuvant to medical treatment.

Expressivity and the meaning of melody

Despite various studies about meaningful music therapeutic interventions in the treatment of cancer, there are no specific recommendations about the expressivity of patients during musical improvisations, whether rhythmically, melodically, or harmonically oriented. In addition there is little written about the way in which women express themselves in music therapy in relation to the therapist. Creative music therapy, an approach that actively pulls the client into the process of performing music – the therapeutic gestalt – exerts an influence on the abilities of the patient to express herself (Aldridge 1996).

Expression is an important aspect of musical improvisation and can appear in various forms of musical parameters. If expressivity is an important aspect in the treatment of breast cancer, and melody is an important form of musical expression in our modern culture, then it makes sense to develop the melodic playing of patients in music therapy. Melodic improvisation offers possibilities to bring the problematic aspect of expressivity in breast cancer patients into an artistic context. Such improvisation may provide women with the opportunity to find their own individual form of expression.

Melody is an important aspect of musical expression, it is related to inner experiences and memory, and can function as an intimate companion along the various paths of one's life. Melody has been, and still is, the most familiar and widely disseminated aspect of music during all periods of time and in all cultures. It is the element of music that provides not only the common quality of music but also reveals the composer's artistic skills. It is hardly possible to answer why some melodies appeal to us more than others, why some melodies continue to live in us, and why we eventually tire of others.

Melody is an independent *tone-movement* that unfolds itself in the matrix of time and is distinguished from other less independent sequences of tones by its inner logical consistency, or vocalisability, or easy comprehensibility, or by firmness and unity of its gestalt, and includes the element of rhythm in its concrete expression. Aspects of form and gestalt may be completed by attributes of self-sufficiency, self-containment, structure, organization, singability, monodism and catchiness. Such adjectival expressions are found in common language as 'melodic', 'tuneful', or 'melodious'.

Besides these attributes, two other expectations are seen as important aspects of melody; *originality* and *expressivity*. Besides the elements of evenness, symmetry and convention, a proportional contribution of novelty and surprise must be present (Abraham and Dahlhaus 1982). It is this factor of expressivity that is of vital importance for women who have had a breast removed.

Expressivity, too, emerges from Hegel's aesthetic implying that the human being can best express her inner world, her soul, through melody and in doing so, simultaneously releases herself from the bonds of suffering or enjoyment (Abraham and Dahlhaus 1982). For Hegel, the inner self of the human being is not only absorbed in itself but at the same time is able to stand beside itself. By experiencing a feeling both present and distant at the same time, a releasing effect may arise. Hegel sees this double characteristic of feeling (emphatic and distant at the same time), as justified in the determinable connection between melody and rhythm and the tonal harmonic of the 17th to 19th century. He emphasises the essential melodic elements: rhythm and harmony, the rules and structures of which are important for melody. Their significance for melody is that they are supports on which melody can stand in order to unfold itself and not to pass into formless shapes.

Important aspects for music therapy

These historical, theoretical and cultural perspectives of music are of significance in that they offer a coherent frame to view the meaning of melodic improvisation within the therapeutic context. In using music as a form of creative therapy, the individual is not only engaged as a perceiving and experiencing person, but is also involved as an acting person. Between perception and experience we find that which is produced, the actual material of performed music.

There is no point in concentrating on rules, regulations or normative melodic constructions, when we are looking for the typical elements of melody. What matters is that we concentrate on separate single melodic elements and attempt to catch the effect of how they are acting in combination. These elements, coming out of the patients creative process as something new and consisting of a rhythmic and melodic cell or motif, may have a connection to harmonic structure and dynamic variables which can be discovered in the music (Aldridge 1998).

Therapeutically, it means that we are able to continually look afresh at the musical material, to discover the particular ways in which clients choose to express themselves in order to find their own appropriate form of expression. If melody reflects expressivity, which itself relieves suffering, then we would be advised to pursue the development of melodic motifs. As these motifs are based upon rhythm and harmony, to maintain expressive form, then we must consider the musical improvisation as a whole. To develop melody then, a substantive harmonic and rhythmic base must be achieved. This can be accomplished by the use of several tuned percussive instruments that are available for melodic improvisation; metallophone, xylophone, chime bars, glockenspiel, marimbaphone and vibraphone. By the horizontal arrangement of the individual tones a priori, playing movement is given which correlates with spatial tone distances of small and big. The very spatial structure of the playing surface proposes melodic forms.

The musical structure that facilitates a melodic expression may be seen as isomorphic with that of the creative musical relationship which facilitates expression and encourages the relief of suffering.

Case study

I would like to present an example of melodic improvisation with a 35-year-old woman in the week immediately following the operation for the removal of her left breast and surrounding tissue. My intention is to demonstrate that melody holds opportunities for the patient to find her own individual form of expression, although she had no musical background other than school music. She did however enjoy music.

The therapist's creative therapeutic approach is based on a method, initially developed for mentally, emotionally and physically handicapped children by Nordoff and Robbins (1977). This method has been recently extended to work with adult patients. An emphasis is made on the creatively improvised musical playing of patient and therapist together, using a variety of percussion drums, congas, cymbals, templeblocks, metallophone, xylophone, vibraphone and sometimes string instruments.

The music therapy sessions with breast cancer patients in general occurs during the immediate post-operative, inpatient phase of two to three weeks. The sessions take place twice a week with a duration of about thirty minutes per session. Some of the women also undergo radiation therapy as well as chemotherapy.

Despite the small amount of music therapy sessions that were available to the patients, it became clear to the therapist what an important role music therapy played during the post-operative phase, immediately after a mastectomy (the removal of a breast) or part-resection (the removal of part of the breast). At a time when there were many mixed and powerful emotions, music therapy provided the ability to bring creatively those emotions into an expressive form within the context of a personal relationship. Some patients expressed themselves on different instruments with intensity and violence, often followed by crying. The therapist had the impression that there was not only an urgent need for expression, but also a struggle to establish a new identity was taking place. Melody played a meaningful role within the therapeutic process. In playing an improvised melody patients experienced a new world of expression. These experiences, which emerged from their melodic playing, were deep and enabled them to cope with their momentarily difficult and burdening situation.

During my work with breast cancer patients, three questions have become important for my work as a music therapist. How does the client develop her melodic playing in the context of musical improvisation? What are the relevant nuances of her emotional expressivity and their relationship to the melody she plays? What does it mean for the client to express herself through the nature of melody?

The following example is an improvisational part of the sixth session with a breast cancer patient, who was in her early-rehabilitation phase after the removal of a breast.

Figures 10.1 to 10.4 follow one another, whereas Figures 10.5 and 10.6 derive from a later section of the improvisation course.

Instruments

Patient: Metallophone, register of the tonal part: c1 – A flat2,
             c-minor harmonic scale

Therapist: piano

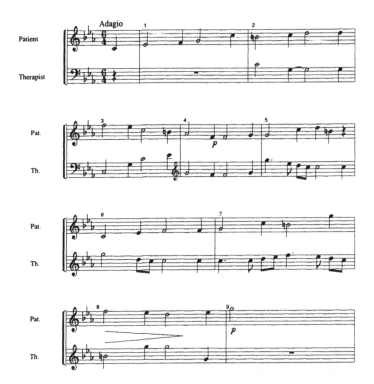

Figure 10.1

The example begins on an upbeat. A rhythmic cell is recognisable. You may see it like the shoot of a plant that in itself has the possibility to develop. It is known that the rhythms are ordered like the ancient system of the verse form; the metrical foot. In the ancient world, the patients chosen rhythm would be described as an iambic foot. This rhythmical cell is meaningful because it holds the patient within her active playing, gives her a grip on herself and offers her enough stability to discover the melodic component and, at the same time, it is a moving impulse leading her into the tonal space of the c-minor scale, which also leads into the harmonic field of c-minor.

From my experience it is a sense of rhythm which allows a sense of melody. As the patient has chosen the form of a metrical foot, it may be seen like a 'way of walking' that is leading her through the improvisation and setting the tone for the rest of the improvisation.

To summarise: Figure 10.1 is an orientation to the c-minor harmonic field. The patient starts on the tonic keynote and naturally finds her way, passing the fifth to the octave and higher fourth. After the first four bars, as therapist, I bring in the melodic element to change this orientation to one of dynamic movement and flexibility associated with melody.

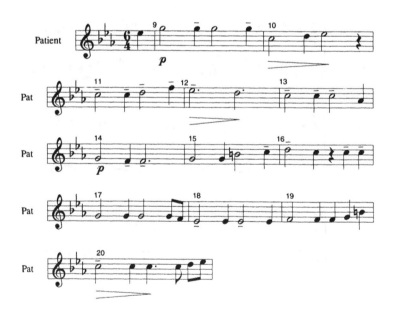

Figure 10.2

In Figure 10.2, we no longer see an orientation to the given c-minor tones. She is consciously listening, which is apparent in her delicate touch. She is perceiving the tonal space harmonically. She accentuates some central tones: the tonic keynote and the fifth. Her harmonic experience is strengthened by playing in a homophonic way. The patient has chosen oriented fixed notes within the tonal space – she starts from these tones by repeating them and goes back to them. When the piano part (which was in the background) comes into the foreground with a melody, she plays a harmonic middle-part. In the last bar the patient comes in with an upbeat melodic figure. This leads to Figure 10.3.

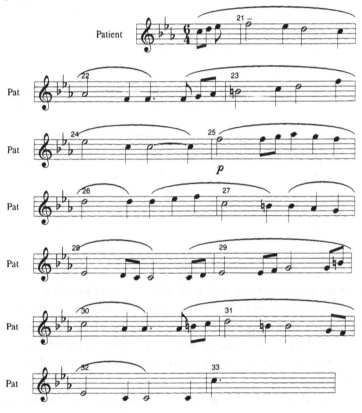

Figure 10.3

The patient herself gives a melodic form to her improvised playing. The structure of the pitch is in the foreground. The pitch is formed and at the same time she develops a rhythmical variety. Both melodic and rhythmic

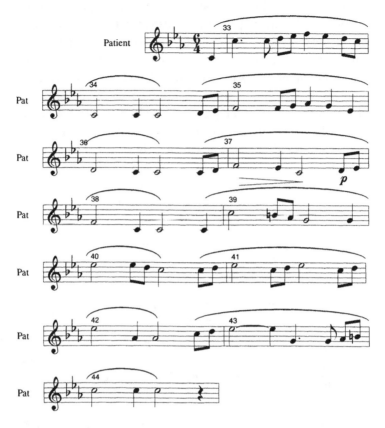

Figure 10.4

elements are corresponding with each other, they are building a symbiosis with one another. One note is related to another as indicated by the slurs.

We can see in this example the development of formal principles of musical composition; the building of two bar phrases, a melodic structure, a tonal orientation returning to the keynote and an experiential element of music played as form.

In Figure 10.4, a more shaped melodic line appears. It starts with an upbeat octave leap, followed by ascending and descending tones, which are formed in two bar phrases. Consequently, the patient makes the tonic keynote audible.

In Figure 10.5, the patient stresses the beginning of the bar that facilitates the descending scale movement. In Figure 10.6, she varies this scale movement in horizontal direction around the central tones of the harmonic minor scale.

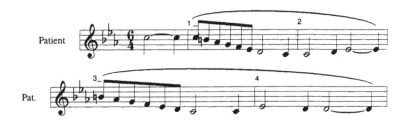

Figures 10.5

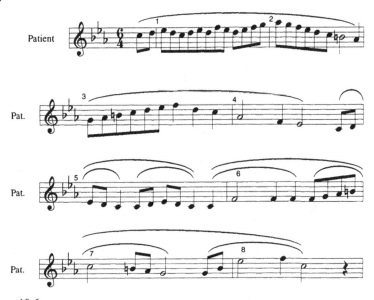

Figure 10.6

Looking at the melody-movement of her playing in more detail there are typical forms of motifs that arise out of the first exposed rhythmic cell (see Figure 10.7). In measures 28–29 she is building sequences of a motif in an upward movement. In measures 40–42 she is giving the motif more importance by repeating it. It is possible to recognise a corresponding melodic construction which often encircles four bars. The harmonic frame, offered by the therapist, takes on the aesthetic musical foundation over which the patients melodic improvisation can develop freely.

The examples show the ability of the patient to express herself melodically. Her comments on this experience was that: 'She had had a

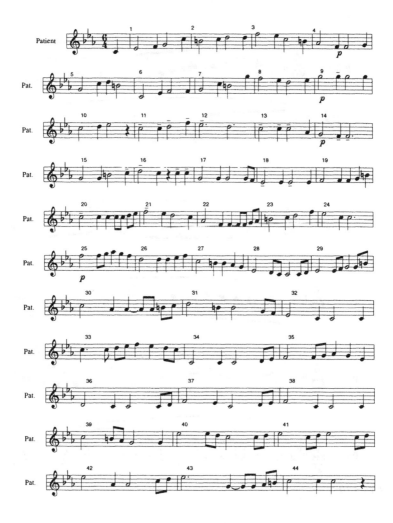

Figure 10.7

wonderful walk through the sunny streets of Paris.' This made me think of the way she began her improvisation (see Figure 10.1), with the classical form of an iambic foot, as a chosen 'way of walking'. The 'walking' led her, step by step, through the improvisation, and set the tone for the following melodic development.

As for the nuances of the patients emotional expressivity, we see them in the way she combines the elements of rhythm, tension of tone, tone colour, harmony, articulation, phrase and form, and the way that she is able to feel and express herself aesthetically through these elements. This musical expressivity, the gradual development of flowing melodic movement, and the continuing creation of newly arising sequences of tones indicate that the patient, in experiencing the musical elements, develops a flexibility that is supported and held by the harmonic structure offered by the therapist.

The harmonic structure with its strong expressiveness of tension and relaxation contributes to a deeper melodic experience. As the harmonic framework, especially from Figure 10.3 onwards, is taken over increasingly and maintained by the therapist it may be seen as a 'prime pattern', or 'prototype' of tonal confirmation that supports and holds the patients melodic playing. It may be that the given c-minor harmonic scale, with the causing tension of intrinsic semitones and the augmented second between the sixth and seventh tone, is a trigger for the freely unfolding melodic playing. The inherent tone tension of the scale could have given rise to the kinetic energy and vitality which is shown in her playing. Each tone is placed in a certain balance of strength and tension to the other, and that is articulated and played with different touch. The client is giving each tone a functional meaning for the overall melodic course (see Figures 10.4, 10.5 and 10.6). Because of the lively character of the playing, it is not possible to eliminate the emotional quality of the patient's playing from the musical material created by her. It is this fusion of expressivity and musical material that rises above the transient and incidental occurrence of tone sequences. What, in the moment of creation, seems to be incidental becomes for the patient meaningful.

The experience of an unfolding melody is an experience of wholeness, a gestalt, a creation that possesses more features than the sum of its single elements would make up. The qualities of the *melodic gestalt* are demonstrated by the concreteness of its form, the synthesis of its single elements and its possibility for transposition into other registers. Looking at the relation to harmony in the clients playing, especially to the basic tone, we may presume that the patient has discovered a way of expression that on one hand centres on herself and on the other hand offers her a reorientation towards herself.

In terms of therapeutic value, the melodic improvisation indicates that the patient has found a form with which she can express herself. This can be seen in her ability to combine and balance the elements of rhythm, pitch, tension of tones, harmony, phrasing and form; her ability to express freely through these elements; and her relationship to harmony as shown by her orientation to the basic tone. Developing a melodic theme supports her need for expression, providing the possibilities to feel and create in her own unique way. She experiences her own creative energy as performed in a time structure that is oriented to her needs. Within the context of the therapeutic relationship, she has the possibility to experience herself in a spontaneous and authentic way. My proposition is that she is encouraged to establish a new identity that is aesthetic and that provides a new orientation in her life. Perhaps the value of the basic tone that frequently is picked up by the patient is that it anchors this new identity and provides a basis for a new orientation.

Conclusion

We know that cancer is a complex disease demanding psychological, emotional and social considerations moving away from a one-sided medical treatment of symptoms that reduces women to   passive medical objects. While numerous authors correlate a cancer personality with the suppression of emotion, physical inactivity, aggression instead of certainty and a lack of flexibility in changing behaviour, music therapy appears to encourage the very opposite. Flexibility in playing leading to the certainty of melodic expression, itself indicative of a emotional articulacy, are characteristics of this case example. Perhaps we need to reflect upon the cultural circumstances under which women are challenged to express themselves when challenged by a disfiguring, and potentially lethal, disease. It may not be their coping mechanisms that are inappropriate, but our ways of understanding their needs that are lacking.

Through melody, the woman in this study, finds a way to put her feelings and musical intuition into action. Her creative energy is dynamically challenged and brought into an expressive form that makes sense to her. Expressivity, shown in this way, reflects the process of emotional recovery and points the way to a new identity. For breast cancer patients, faced with expressing overwhelming feelings, challenged with adjusting to a new, radically altered, future, the process of bringing their feelings into conscious form without any immediate verbal label, may be a significant step on the road to recovery.

For this woman it was enough for her to comment on the last improvisation, that is was like a walk through the sunny streets of Paris. As this is music therapy, and not psychotherapy, there was no imperative for any further verbalisation. What had been stated was in the music. The art form was the expressive form, it sufficed as it stood alone. Of course, if the woman had wanted to talk further about her experiences with the therapist, the opportunities were there for discussion and analysis. Simply exhorting women to express themselves, when that is the very problem itself, is futile. Encouraging the expression of anger may indeed be carthartic, but in the longer term may not be subtle enough or positive, enough for prolonged recovery. Music therapy offers a means of expression that attaches no value labels. Each woman is inspired to create her own expressions in her own time. She is given the opportunity to accept herself in a spontaneous authentic way, she creates an identity that is aesthetic. In the therapeutic relationship, this is fostered as a form that is aesthetic not moral. She performs, she is not judged. Her inner realities are experienced as beautiful (Aldridge, Brandt and Wohler 1990).

Active, creative music therapy is an intervention that offers a chance for clients to use their own creativity and creative strength to cope with their crisis and maintain coherence throughout the illness. In this way, it is possible to find a different musical form appropriate to the varying stages of the disease, whether they be to recovery or through the accompaniment to dying.

If we look at Benzon's structure of musical development within a culture referred to earlier, we see how the harmonic structure of the music provides the architecture of the therapeutic relationship. Within this architecture, we hear how the woman first develops a forward movement based upon a simple rhythmic cell; the 'iambic foot'. She later refers to her 'Walk through Paris'. From the stability of a rhythmic impetus, that she herself has made, this develops into rhythmic phrasing. The melodic motif, based upon the rhythmical figure, expands into a melodic line. Not only is this leading in the musical form, she is also leading in the relationship and developing a new expressive identity. Personal expressivity occurs within a culturally accepted form. Music therapy also allows an architecture for finding a new personal identity within a social context that is itself valid and meaningful within a given cultural context.

CHAPTER 11

Writing and Therapy
Into a New Tongue

Rob Finlayson

I am the poet of the Body and the poet of the Soul,
The pleasures of heaven are with me and the pains of hell are with me,
The first I graft and increase upon myself, the latter I translate into a new
tongue. (Walt Whitman's *Song of Myself*)

'Why do you write?' I once asked a friend.

'For salvation,' was his reply.

There is plenty of anecdotal evidence over the centuries that writing what
you feel and think – and reading what others have written – can alleviate
distress, lift despair, and help to forge a new direction for your life. And, more
and more, writing is being used by therapists as a valuable tool in the healing
process.

Some clinical studies (Pennebaker, Kiecolt-Glaser and Glaser 1988) have
indicated a connection between disclosure of trauma, through written as well
as oral means, and an increase in the body's immune system response. More
research needs to be carried out but, meanwhile, writing is used by therapists
within clinical and psychiatric settings as well as within situations open to the
general public, with people who want to understand their lives better. In the
sections that follow, all of the therapeutic modalities mentioned are used as
adjuncts to the therapist's own modality, except narrative therapy, which
integrates different forms of writing into the therapeutic process, based on a
comprehensive theoretical approach.

Narrative therapy

The narrative therapy of Michael White and David Epston makes use of written language in forms such as invitations, references, certificates, predictions and declarations (White and Epston 1990). Karl Tomm (1990), writing about the pair's work, argues a point that also holds true for all therapy which uses writing:

> ... the single most important domain that White has opened is that of 'externalising the problem'. When the distinction of the problem can be clearly separated from the distinction of the person, it becomes possible to carefully examine the dynamics and direction of the interaction between persons and problems ...(p.7)

This 'externalisation' process which written forms can make so clear, occurs whether what is written is a simple list or a poem containing complex metaphor and rhythm. The power of writing a few words can bring about a revelation or disclosure that assists the therapeutic process. Schloss and Grundy (1994) give an example of how poetry – both hearing other's and writing your own – can assist people to bring issues to light. The example is from what they call a 'sociopoetic' pattern (because of its similarity to sociodrama) of a group therapy which utilises writing, taken from their work with several hundred groups:

> In another group in which *Tree at My Window* (Lathem 1969) was read, a member said he liked Frost's image of the tree concerned with outer weather and of the narrator concerned with inner weather. The member said he had not only inner weather, but a whole inner landscape of situations, events, and some personal qualities he rarely spoke about. Another member referred to a book, *The Me Nobody Knows* (Joseph 1969), saying she had always felt like a stranger with others, even people in the group, because she had never shown who she really was. The leader suggested that members write a poem exploring the 'me nobody knows' and express at least one part of themselves which they rarely showed to another. These pieces were read aloud. Some revealed childhood indiscretions. A professional man admitted that he enjoyed cooking, but felt people would laugh at him or think he was effeminate. (Schloss and Grundy 1994, p.93)

Stubbs (1980) proposes that a society with a writing system has 'new intellectual resources which greatly facilitate thought', in that:

(1) Each generation no longer has to begin from scratch or from what the previous generation can remember and pass on.

(2) Writing allows for the accumulation of recorded wisdom.

(3) Writing enables findings to be recorded in a form that makes them easier to study and consider critically, and this in turn leads to more discoveries.

(4) The information content of written language is higher and less predictable.

(5) Writing dramatically transforms the teacher-student relationship and promotes independence in thought, as there can be knowledge without a knower, existing independently in books. (p.107)

'Recourse to the written tradition in therapy', state White and Epston (1990, p.35), 'promotes the formalisation, legitimation, and continuity of local popular knowledge, the independent authority of persons, and the creation of a context for the emergence of new discoveries and possibilities'.

To give a simple example, there can be a considerable sense of personal achievement in writing in a form never before attempted. A terminally ill man in a day-hospice group with which I worked approached me after a group poetry writing session. He had spent his working life on merchant ships and then mine sites and, today, had written his first poem. He said:

> I don't want to sound as if I'm grateful for this cancer, but I've done some things because of it that I never would've dreamed of, like writing a poem. I tell you, this is wonderful!

He had written, after the group had been discussing relationships with nature:

> The sea lit up
> with phosphorous
> whilst travelling
> thru rivers
> in the archipelago.
>
> The crowd was excited
> in anticipation
> of what lay ahead,
> of wine, woman and song.

He died a few weeks later.

Poetry therapy

Poetry, specifically, is used in therapeutic contexts in various ways. Fox describes the workings of poetry-as-therapy thus: 'Poetry provides guidance, revealing what you didn't know you knew before you wrote or read the poem. This moment of surprising yourself with your own words of wisdom or of being surprised by the poems of others is at the heart of poetry as healer.' (Fox 1997, p.3)

Poetry can clarify seemingly inexpressible feelings and draw together seemingly unrelated events and feelings. From a conversation with a terminally ill woman, I composed the following poem, based entirely on her own words. This is a simple technique which I call 'reflective autobiography'. It is particularly useful with people who are too ill to write themselves.

The Door

A Conversation[1]

I'm not afraid
of death
It's like going
through a door
But mine's stuck
and I need
the carpenter
to come along
and fix it
I've done most
of the work
of getting ready
to meet my Maker
That takes
quite a bit of thought
because sometimes

1 Rob Finlayson

to make good
can upset people
I think everything's
done now
except for one thing:
it's my son's birthday
and I forgot to ring him

How does poetry 'work'? What makes poetry a useful tool in therapy? Charles Ansell (1978) argues that the 'mind' of the poet is both open and empty. It is open to free introspection, open to direct communication with his unconscious and empty of distractions of those anxieties that propel most of us into preformed modes of thinking and feeling. Buber hints at this necessary frame of mind, open to the novel and empty of the 'preconcerted', if human encounter is to be creative. The ego state after a thoroughgoing psychoanalysis may be said to be free of the anxieties that life sets down on our path.

The associative techniques of metaphor and assonance can link disparate themes in a person's life. Words used in this way can become more consciously powerful or serve as delicate indicators of difficult issues. For example, the following poem by Anne Harrington uses one strong image to talk about emotions.

Jammed / Crammed / Damned [2]

Emotions piled in a corner
   One on top of another
   Stuffed in
   Crammed
   Jammed
   Heaped high
   Overlooked
   Too busy to get to
Like days' old – or is it years' old – laundry
in a too-small hamper.
   Smelly

2   Anne Harrington

Soiled
Discarded
Embarrassing
   A blight in an otherwise well-ordered room.

The lid won't shut.
I cram them in.
A few spill onto the floor
   A stray grey
   A raging red
   A simmering burnt orange
   A withholding white

Don't mix the colors with the whites.
Wash in cold water.
Do not add bleach.
Warranted to reveal manufacturer's defects.

Emotions, mostly contained, put away.
Waiting. Over there. In the corner.

Journal writing

Journal writing has been used by many therapists and, increasingly, educators, to encourage patients and students to express their thoughts and feelings. One participant in a journal workshop on loss and grief, wrote that the most useful part of the workshop, for her, was 'getting in touch with my feelings and then writing to that feeling; realising where I could really help myself' (personal communication).

Anais Nin, one of the world's most famous journal keepers, describes writing a journal or 'diarising' with a colleague (in Rainier 1978, p.9) as an exercise in creative will; as an exercise in synthesis; as a means to create a world according to our wishes, not those of others; as a means of creating the self, of giving birth to ourselves. Diary writing is taught as a way of reintegrating ourselves when experience shatters us, to help us out of silence and the anxieties of alienation.

Nursing education, in some schools, adopts reflective journal writing as a way of integrating the scientific methodology of nursing practice with the feelings, thoughts and personal behaviours of the student. It aims to encourage self-directed learning. Both the clinical nurse educator and the nursing student can benefit from using a reflective journal as a learning tool. Learning occurs as journal writing connects the student with self, faculty, other learners, nursing and health care systems. Furthermore, reflective journal writing enhances the use of self-analysis and critical thinking; reinforces the importance of utilising theory to guide nursing practice; and establishes a co-operative educator-student relationship built on a model of mentorship (Riley-Doucet and Wilson 1997).

Journal writing can be focused on specific events or emotions. For example, one writer keeps a 'happy' journal in which she records only happy thoughts, feelings and events in order to encourage that emotion in her life. I host 'Grief Journal' workshops for bereaved people and palliative care staff, and 'Self-Care Journal' workshops for staff. Feedback from the 'Grief Journal' workshops consistently indicates feelings of well-being and catharsis after the day's work. The 'Self-Care Journal' workshops are in strong demand from staff throughout Australia.

Conclusion

Entering the world of the professional writer enables the therapist to make use of the craft's techniques for therapeutic ends. Poetry, narrative, journal writing are a few of the techniques available.

We are the stories we tell ourselves. If we learn how to tell them so that the ones we no longer find useful are less important, then we can begin to free ourselves, to 'rewrite' our lives and become authors with the power to create our *healthy* stories.

References

Aasgaard, T. (1996a) 'Musikkterapi som livskvalitetsfremmende faktor i kreftomsorgen.' ('Music therapy promoting quality of life in cancer care.') *Kreftsykepleie 12*, 1, 6–7.

Aasgaard, T. (1996b) 'Musikkterapi til barn med kreft, del 2: noen yeblikks fristunder fra en vond hverdag.' ('Music therapy for children with cancer, part 2: moments of freedom during a hard time.') *Musikkterapi 21*, 4, 29–38.

Abraham, L. and Dahlhaus, C. (1982) *Melodielehre.* Wiesbaden: Laaber-Verlag.

Aldridge, D. (1987a) 'Families, cancer and dying.' *Family Practice 4*, 212–218.

Aldridge, D. (1987b) 'A team approach to terminal care: personal implications for patients and practitioners.' *Journal of the Royal College of General Practitioners 37*, 364.

Aldridge, D. (1987c). *One Body: A Guide to Healing in the Church.* London: S.P.C.K.

Aldridge, D. (1989) 'Research strategies in a hospital setting.' *Complementary Medical Research 3*, 2, 20–24.

Aldridge, D. (1993) 'Hope, meaning and the creative art therapies in the treatment of AIDS.' *The Arts in Psychotherapy 20*, 285–297.

Aldridge, D. (1996) *Music Therapy Research and Practice in Medicine: From Out of the Silence.* London: Jessica Kingsley Publishers.

Aldridge, D and Verney, R. (1988) 'Research in a hospital setting.' *Holistic Health 18*, 9–10.

Aldridge, D., Brandt, G. and Wohler, D. (1990) 'Toward a common language among the creative art therapies.' *The Arts in Psychotherapy 17*, 3, 189–195.

Aldridge, G (1996) '"A walk through Paris": the development of melodic expression in music therapy with a breast-cancer patient.' *The Arts in Psychotherapy 23*, 207–223.

Aldridge, G. (1998) The development of melody in the context of improvised music therapy with melodic examples: 'A walk through Paris' and 'The Farewell melody'. Unpublished doctoral thesis. Aalborg University, Denmark.

Alexander, D. (1993) 'Psychological/social research.' In D. Doyle, G. Hanks and N. Macdonald (eds) *Oxford Textbook of Palliative Medicine.* Oxford: Oxford University Press.

Ansdell, G. (1995) *Music for Life: Aspects of Creative Music Therapy with Adults.* London: Jessica Kingsley Publishers.

Ansell, C. (1978) 'Psychoanalysis and poetry.' In A. Lerner (ed) *Poetry in the Therapeutic Experience.* Saint Louis: MMB.

Auden, W. (1948) 'Criticism in a mass society.' *The Mint 1*, 13.

Bailey, L. (1983) 'The effects of live music versus tape-recorded music on hospitalized cancer patients.' *Music Therapy 3*, 1, 17–28.

Bailey, L. (1984) 'The use of songs with cancer patients and their families.' *Music Therapy 4*, 1, 5–17.

Bailey, L. (1985) 'The role of music therapy.' In M.O.C. Pain (ed) *Syllabus of the Postgraduate Course.* New York: Memorial Sloan-Kettering Cancer Center.

Bailey, L. (1986) 'Music therapy in pain management.' *Journal of Pain Symptom Management 1*, 1, 25–8.

Bakhtiar, L. (1976) *Sufi: Expressions of the Mystic Quest*. London: Thames and Hudson.

Beggs, C. (1991) 'Life review with a palliative care patient.' In K. Bruscia (ed) *Case studies in Music Therapy*. Phoenixville, PA: Barcelona Publishers.

Benzon, W. (1993) 'The United States of the blues: on the crossing of African and European cultures in the 20th century.' *Journal of Social and Evolutionary Systems 16*, 4, 401–438.

Berti, L., Hoffmann, S. and Möbus, V. (1993) 'Traditioneller vs. "modifizierter" forschungsansatz im rahmen psychoonkologischer studien.' *Psychotherapie, Psychosomatik und Medizinische Psychologie 43*, 151–158.

Bonny, H. (1978) GIM Monograph #2. *The Role of Taped Music programs in the GIM Process*. Baltimore: ICM Press.

Brandt, M. (1996) '"This is my life". Songwriting and song interpretation with Huntington's patients.' *'Sound and Psyche' 8th Congress of Music Therapy*. Hamburg, 216.

Brodsky, W. (1989) 'Music therapy as an intervention for children with cancer in isolation rooms.' First International Paediatric Oncology Nursing Meeting (Israel 1987, Jerusalem). *Music Therapy 8*, 1, 17–34.

Bruscia, K. (1991a) *Case Studies in Music Therapy*. Phoenixville, Philadelphia: Barcelona Publishers.

Bruscia, K. (1991b) 'Embracing life with AIDS: psychotherapy through guided imagery and music (GIM).' In K. Bruscia (ed) *Case Studies in Music Therapy*. Phoenixville, Philadelphia: Barcelona Publishers.

Bruscia, K. (1995) 'Images in AIDS.' In C. Lee (ed) *Lonely Waters*. Oxford: Sobell Publications.

Bunt, L. (1994) *Music Therapy: An Art Beyond Words*. London: Routledge and Kegan Paul.

Butler, R. and Lewis, M. (1982) *Ageing and Mental Health*. St. Louis, MO: C.V. Mosby and Co.

Byock, I. (1994) 'When suffering persists...' *Journal of Palliative Care 10*, 2, 8–13.

Campbell, D. (1997) *The Mozart Effect*. New York: Avon Books.

Cantacuzino, M. (1993) *Till Break of Day: Meeting the Challenge of HIV and AIDS at London Lighthouse*. London: Heinemann.

Carpenter, R. and Bettis, J. (1973) *Yesterday Once More*. Hollywood, CA: Almo Music Corps/Sweet Harmony Music/Hanner and Nails Music.

Carter, B. (1993). 'Long-term survivors of breast cancer. A qualitative descriptive study.' *Cancer Nursing 16*, 5, 354–361.

Carter, B. (1994) 'Surviving breast cancer. A problematic work re-entry.' *Cancer Practice 2*, 2, 135–140.

Carter, R. and Carter, C (1993). 'Individual and marital adjustment in spouse pairs subsequent to mastectomy.' *American Journal of Family Therapy 21*, 4, 291–300.

Carter, R. Carter, C. and Prosen, H. (1992) 'Emotional and personality types of breast cancer patients and spouses.' *The American Journal of Family Therapy 20*, 4, 300–308.

Connell, H. (1989) 'Promoting self-expression.' *Nursing Times 85*, 15, 52–54.

Curtis, S. (1986) 'The effect of music on pain relief and relaxation of the terminally ill.' *Journal of Music Therapy 23*, 10–24.

Crossley, N. (1994) 'Merleau-Ponty, the elusive body and carnal sociology.' *Body and Society 1*, 1, 43–63.

Curtis, S. (1987) 'Music therapy: a positive approach in Huntington's Disease.' *Proceedings of the 13th National Conference of the Australian Music Therapy Association.* Melbourne: Australian Music Therapy Association, Inc.

Dawes, S. (1985a) 'Case study: advanced stage Huntington's Disease.' In Chiu and Teltscher (eds) *Handbook for Caring in Huntington's Disease.* Melbourne: Arthur Preston Centre Huntington's Disease Unit Clinc.

Dawes, S. (1985b) The role of music therapy in caring in Huntington's Disease. In Chiu and Teltscher (eds) *Handbook for Caring in Huntington's Disease.* Melbourne: Arthur Preston Centre Huntington's Disease Clinic.

Delmonte, I-I. (1993) 'Why work with the dying.' In C. Lee (ed) *Lonely Waters.* Oxford: Sobell House.

Doyle, D., Hanks, G. and Macdonald, N. (1993) *Oxford Textbook of Palliative Medicine.* Oxford: Oxford University Press.

Dreyfus, H. (1987) 'Foucault's critique of psychiatric medicine.' *The Journal of Medicine and Philosophy 12,* 311–333.

Durham C. (1995) 'Music therapy with severely head-injured clients.' In C. Lee (ed) *Lonely Waters.* Oxford: Sobell House.

Erdonmez, D. (1976) 'The effect of music therapy in the treatment of Huntington's Chorea patients.' *Proceedings of the 2nd National Conference of the Australian Music Therapy Association.* N.S.W.: Australian Music Therapy Association, Inc.

Erdonmez, D. (1995) 'A journey of transition with guided imagery and music.' In C. Lee (ed) *Lonely waters.* Oxford: Sobell House 125–134.

Fagen, T. (1982) 'Music therapy in the treatment of anxiety and fear in terminal pediatric patients.' *Music Therapy 2,* 1, 13–23.

Feld, S. (1990) *Sound and Sentiment: Birds, Weeping, Poetics and Song in Kaluli Expression.* Philadelphia: University of Pennsylvania Press.

Fiddes, P. (1988) *The Creative Suffering of God.* London: Clarendon Paperbacks.

Fischer, N. (1997) 'Frankfurt School Marxism and the ethical meaning of art: Herbert Marcuse's *The Aesthetic Dimension.' Communication Theory 7,* 4, 362–381.

Fischer, N (1996) 'From aesthetic education to environmental aesthetics.' *CLIO 25,* 4, 365–391.

Folstein, S. (1989) *Huntington's Disease: A Disorder of Families.* London: The John Hopkins University Press.

Forinash, M. (1990) *The Phenomenology of Music Therapy with the Terminally Ill.* Ann Arbor: University Microfilms, 91–02617.

Fox, J. (1997) *Poetic Medicine.* Putnam, NY: Jeremy P. Tarcher.

Frampton, D.R. (1986) 'Restoring creativity to the dying patient.' *Br-Med-J-Clin-Res 293,* 6562, 1593–5.

Froehlich, M.-A. (1984) 'A comparison of the effect of music therapy and medical play therapy as the verbalization behavior of pediatric patients.' *Journal of Music Therapy 21,* 1, 2–15.

Froehlich, M.-A. (1996) 'Music therapy with the terminally ill child.' In M.-A. Froehlich (ed) *Music Therapy with Hospitalized Children.* Cherry Hill, NJ: Jeffrey Books.

Geyer, S. (1993) 'Life events, chronic difficulties and vulnerability factors preceding breast cancer.' *Social Science and Medicine, 37,* 12, 1545–1555.

Glaser, B and Strauss, A. (1967) *The Discovery of Grounded Theory*. Chicago: Aldine.

Gregory, D. (1994) 'The myth of control: suffering in palliative care.' *Journal of Palliative Care 10*, 2, 18–22.

Greisinger, A., Lorimor, R., Aday, L., Winn, R. and Baile, W. (1997) 'Terminally ill cancer patients. Their most important concerns.' *Cancer Practice 5*, 3, 147–154.

Grenzel, H. and Binzack, T. (1995) 'Die behandlung schwerkraner u. sterbender in einer klinishcen hospizeinrichtung.' *Das Krankenhaus 11*, 536–543.

Griessmeier, B. and Bossinger, W. (1994) *Musiktherapie mit Krebskranken Kindern*. Stuttgart: Gustav Fisscher Verlag.

Groom, J. and Dawes, S. (1985) 'Enhancing the self-image of people with Huntington's Disease through the use of music, movement and dance.' *Proceedings of the 11th National Conference of the Australian Music Therapy Association Incorporated*. Melbourne: Australian Music Therapy Association, Inc.

Gross, R., Sasson, Y., Zarhy, M. and Zohar, J. (1998) 'Healing environment in psychiatric hospital design.' *General Hospital Psychiatry 20*, 108–114.

Gunzburg, J. (1997) *Healing Through Meeting: Martin Buber's Conversational Approach to Psychotherapy*. London: Jessica Kingsley Publishers.

Gustorff, D. (1990) 'Lieder ohne Worte.' *Musiktherapeutische Umschau 11*, 120–126.

Gustorff, D. (1992a) 'Annehmen und verstehen in der musiktherapie.' In R. Brinker, B. van Hoek and K. Schlaaf-Kirschner (eds) *Annehmen und Verstehen-Förderung von Menschen mit sehr schweren Behinderungen*. Landesverband Nordrhein-Westfalen e.V: Lebenshilfe für geistig Behinderte.

Gustorff, D. (1992b) 'Schöpferische musiktherapie bei schmerzpatienten.' *Der Schmerz 6*, S1, 47–48.

Gustorff, D. (1995) 'Begegnung mit der ältesten leiden der welt-musiktherapie mit einem schmerzpatienten.' In P. Petersen (ed) *'Destruktivität und Heilkraft' 2. Dresdner Symposion für künstlerische Therapien*. Dresden, 31–36.

Gustorff, D. (1996) 'Musiktherapie als orientierungshilfe bei bewußtseinsgestörten patienten.' *Intensiv 2*, 59–61.

Hall, B. (1998) 'Patterns of spirituality in persons with advanced HIV disease.' *Research in Nursing and Health, 21*, 143–153.

Harper, P. (1991) *Huntington's Disease*. London: W.B. Saunders Company Ltd.

Hartley, N. (1994) *In Retrospect, in Prospect: Music Therapy with Those Who Are Living with or Who Are Affected by HIV/AIDS*. Oxford: Sobell House

Herrigel, E. (1988). *The Method of Zen*. London: Penguin Arkana.

Heyde, P. and v. Langsdorff, P. (1983). 'Rehabilitation krebskranker unter einschluß schöpferischer therapien.' *Rehabilitation 22*, 25–27.

Hodder, P. and Turley, A. (1989) *The Creative Option of Palliative Care*. Melbourne: Melbourne Citymission.

Hodges, D and Haack, P. (1996) 'The influence of music on human behavior.' In D. Hodges (ed) *Handbook of Music Psychology*. San Antonio: IMO Press 469–555.

Hogan, B. (1997) *The Experience of Music Therapy for Terminally Ill Patients*. Master of Music, The University of Melbourne, Australia.

Hoskyns, S. (1985) 'Striking the right chord.' *Nursing Mirror,* June 2nd, 14–17.

Hürny, C., Bernhard, J., Bacchi, M., van Wegberg, B., Tomamichel, M., Spek, U., Coates, A., Castiglione, M., Goldhirsch, A. and Senn, J. (1993) 'The Perceived Adjustment to Chronic Illness Scale (PACIS): a global indicator of coping for operable breast cancer patients in clinical trials.' *Support Care Cancer 1*, 200–208.

Janicki, A. (1993) 'Music therapy in Poland.' In C. Maranto (ed) *Music Therapy: International Perspectives.* Pipersville: Jeffrey Books.

Kellehear, A. (1993) *The Unobtrusive Observer: A Guide to Methods.* St. Leonards: Allen and Unwin.

Kenny, C. (1982) *The Mythic Artery.* Atascadero, CA: Ridgeview Publishing Co.

Khan, I. (1983) *The Music of Life.* Santa Fee: Omega Press.

Khan, Sufi Inayat (1979) *The Bowl of Saki.* Geneva: Sufi Publishing Co. Ltd.

Kim, S.H. (1983) *The Nature of Theoretical Thinking in Nursing.* Stamford: Appleton.

Kotarba, J. and Hurt, D. (1995) 'The ethnography of an AIDS hospice: toward a theory of organizational pastiche.' *Symbolic Interaction, 18,* 4 , 413–438.

Kümmel, W.F. (1977) *Musik und Medizin.* Freiburg: Karl Alber.

Lane, D. (1992) 'Music therapy: a gift beyond measure.' *Oncology Nursing Forum 19,* 6, 863–867.

Lathem, E. (1969) *The Poetry of Robert Frost.* New York: Holt, Rinehart and Winston.

Lee, C.A. (1989) 'Structural analysis of therapeutic improvisatory music.' *Journal of British Music Therapy 3,* 2, 11–19.

Lee, C. (1992) The analysis of therapeutic improvisatory music with people living with the HIV virus and AIDS. Unpublished doctoral dissertation. City University, London.

Lee, C. (1995) *Lonely Waters.* Oxford: Sobell House.

Lee, C. (1996) *Music at the Edge: The Music Therapy Experiences of a Musician with AIDS.* London: Routledge.

Lengdobler, H. and Kiessling, W. (1989) 'Gruppenmusiktherapie bei multipler sklerose: ein erster erfahrungsbericht.' ('Group music therapy in multiple sclerosis: initial report of experience.') *Psychother-Psychosom-Med-Psychol. 39,* 9–10, 369–73.

Levine, S. (1982) *Who dies? An Investigation into Conscious Living and Conscious Dying.* New York: Anchor Books.

Lichtenberger, H. (1993) 'Musiktherapie im rahmen der rehabilitation von querschnitt-patienten.' *Praxis Ergo-therapie 6,* 4, 218–222.

Lloyd-Green, L. (1990) 'Music therapy strategies in hospice care.' Unpublished proceedings of the 4th Western Pacific Region of the Medical Women's International Association Conference, Brisbane.

Lochner, C.W. and Stevenson, R.G. (1987) 'Music as a bridge to wholeness. Special issue: cultural and religious perspectives of death.' *Death Studies 12,* 2, 173–180.

Loewy, J. (1997) *Music Therapy and Paediatric Pain.* Cherry Hill, NJ: Jeffrey Books.

Magee, W. (1995a) 'Case studies in Huntington's Disease: music therapy assessment and treatment in the early to advanced stages.' *British Journal of Music Therapy 9,* 2, 13–19.

Magee, W. (1995b) 'Music therapy as part of assessment and treatment for people living with Huntingtons's Disease.' In C. Lee (ed) *Lonely Waters.* Oxford: Sobell House.

Magee, W. (1998) 'Singing My Life, Playing Myself.' Investigating the use of familiar pre-composed music and unfamiliar improvised music in clinical music therapy with individuals with chronic neurological illness. Unpublished doctoral dissertation. University of Sheffield, UK.

Magill Levreault, L. (1993) 'Music therapy in pain and symptom management.' *Journal of Palliative Care 9*, 4, 42–48.

Mahler, M and Benson, D. (1990) 'Cognitive dysfunction in multiple sclerosis: a subcortical dementia?' In S. Rao (ed) *Neurobehavioural Aspects of Multiple Sclerosis.* Oxford: Oxford University Press.

Mandel, S. (1991) 'Music therapy in the hospice: "Musicalive".' *Journal of Palliative Care 9*, 4, 37–39.

Mann, T. (1949) *Doctor Faustus.* London: Minerva.

Maranto, C. (1993) 'Music therapy clinical practice: a global perspective and classification system.' In C. Maranto (ed) *Music Therapy: International Perspectives.* Pipersville: Jeffrey Books.

Marley, L. (1984) 'The use of music with hospitalized infants and toddlers: a descriptive study.' *Journal of Music Therapy 21*, 126–132.

Martin, J. (1989) 'Music therapy in palliative care.' In J. Martin (ed) *The Next Step Forward: Music Therapy with the Terminally Ill.* New York: Calvary Hospital.

Martin, J. (1991) 'Music therapy at the end of life.' In K. Bruscia (ed) *Case Studies in Music Therapy.* Phoenixville, PA: Barcelona Publishers.

Mayr, A. (1985) 'Musik, zeit und gesundheit.' In E. Ruud (ed) *Music and Health.* Oslo: Norsk Musikkforlag.

McCauley, K. (1996) 'Music therapy with pediatric AIDS patients.' In M.-A. Froehlich (ed) *Music Therapy with Hospitalized Children.* Cherry Hill, NJ: Jeffrey Books.

Melamed, B. (1992) 'Family factors predicting children's reactions to anesthesia induction.' In L. Greca, A. Siegel, L. Wallander and C. Walker (eds) *Stress and Coping in Child Health.* New York: The Guilford Press.

Menninger, K. (1959) 'Hope.' *The American Journal of Psychiatry 116*, 12, 481–491.

Morris, M. (1991) 'Psychiatric aspects of Huntington's Disease.' In P. Harper (ed) *Huntington's Disease.* London: W. B. Saunders Company Ltd.

Munro, S. (1984) *Music Therapy in Palliative/Hospice Care.* Saint Louis, MO: MMB.

Munro, S. and Mount, B. (1978) 'Music therapy in palliative care.' *Canadian Medical Association Journal 119*, 9, 1029–34.

Nattiez, J.-J. (1990) *Music and Discourse. Towards a Semiology of Music.* New Jersey: Princeton University Press.

Neugebauer, L. (1993) 'Musik, sinnes- und kindheitsentwicklung.' In H. -D. Decker-Vogt, J. Eschen and W. Mahns (eds) *Kindermusiktherapie.* Bremen: Eres.

Neugebauer, L. (1995) 'Im spannungsfeld zwischen eindruck und ausdruck.' *Das Band 2,* 7–10.

Neugebauer, L. (1998) 'Musik als dialog – eine untersuchung zu physiologischen veränderungen während der musiktherapie.' *Musiktherapeutische Umschau 19*, 29–43.

Nelson, D., Friedman, L., Baer, P., Lane, M. and Smith, F. (1994) 'Subtypes of psychosocial adjustment to breast cancer.' *Journal of Behavioral Medicine, 17*, 2, 127–141.

Nolan, P. (1992) 'Music therapy with bone marrow transplant patients: reaching beyond the symptoms.' In R. Spintge and R. Droh (eds) *Musicmedicine.* Saint Louis: MMB.

Nordoff, P. and Robbins, C. (1977) *Creative Music Therapy.* New York: John Day.

O'Callaghan, C. (1984) 'Musical profiles of dying patients.' *Australian Music Therapy Association Bulletin* 7, 2, 5–11.

O'Callaghan, C. (1989a) 'Isolation in an isolated spot: music therapy in palliative care in Australia.' In J. Martin (ed) *The Next Step Forward: Music Therapy with the Terminally Ill.* New York: Calvary Hospital.

O'Callaghan, C. (1989b) 'The use of music therapists in palliative care.' In P. Hooder and A. Turley (eds) *The Creative Option of Palliative Care.* Melbourne: Melbourne Commission.

O'Callaghan, C. (1990) 'Music therapy skills used in song writing within a palliative care setting.' *Australian Journal of Music Therapy 1*, 15–22.

O'Callaghan, C. (1993) 'Communicating with brain-impaired palliative care patients through music therapy.' *Journal of Palliative Care 9*, 4, 53–55.

O'Callaghan, C. (1994) *Song Writing in Palliative Care.* University of Melbourne, Australia.

O'Callaghan, C. (1996a) 'Lyrical themes in songs written by palliative care patients.' *Journal of Music Therapy 33*, 2, 74–92.

O'Callaghan, C. (1996b) 'Pain, music creativity and music therapy in palliative care.' *Am J Hosp Palliat Care 13*, 2, 43–9.

O'Callaghan, C. and Brown, G. (1989) 'Facilitating communication with brain impaired severely ill people; the impact of music therapy.' *Proceedings of the National Association for Loss and Grief 6th Biennial Conference.* Melbourne: NALAG.

O'Callaghan, C. and Turnbull, G. (1987) 'The application of a neuropsychological knowledge base in the use of music therapy with severely brain damaged, adynamic, multiplesclerosis patients.' *Proceedings of the 13th National Conference of the Australian Music Therapy Association.* Melbourne: AMTA.

Olofsson, A. (1995) 'The value of integrating music therapy and expressive art therapy in working with cancer patients.' In C. Lee (ed) *Lonely Waters: Proceedings of the International Conference Music Therapy in Palliative Care.* Oxford: Sobell House Publications.

Pennebaker, J., Kiecolt-Glaser, J. and Glaser, R. (1988) 'Disclosure of traumas and immune function: Health implications for psychotherapy.' *Journal of Consulting and Clinical Psychology 56*, 239–245.

Pickering, W. (1997) 'Kindness, prescribed and natural, in medicine.' *Journal of Medical Ethics 23*, 2, 116–118.

Porchet Munro, S. (1993) 'Music therapy perspectives in palliative care education.' *Journal of Palliative Care 9*, 4, 39–42.

Rainey Perry, M. (1983) 'Music therapy in the care of Huntington's Disease patients.' *Australian Music Therapy Association Bulletin,* December 6, 3–10.

Rainier, T. (1978) *The New Diary.* Putnam, NY: Jeremy P. Tarcher.

Randall, C. (1982) 'The medical social worker in the rehabilitation team.' In R. Capildeo and A. Maxwell (eds) *Progress In Rehabilitation: Multiple Sclerosis.* London: The Macmillan Press Ltd.

Rawnsley, M. (1994) 'Recurrence of cancer: a crisis of courage.' *Cancer Nursing, 17*, 4, 342–347.

Rees, D. (1991) *Dog Days, White Nights.* London: Third House Publishers.

Riley-Doucet, C. and Wilson, S. (1997) 'A three step method of self-reflection using reflective journal writing.' *Journal of Advanced Nursing 25*, 964–968.

Robbins, C. (1993) 'The creative processes are universal.' In M. Heal and T. Wigram (eds) *Music Therapy in Health and Education.* London: Jessica Kingsley Publishers.

Roy, D. (1997) 'Palliative care: a fragment towards its philosophy.' *Journal of Palliative Care* 13, 1, 3–4.

Salmon, D. (1989) 'Partage: groupwork in palliative care.' In J. Martin (ed) *The Next Step Forward: Music Therapy with the Terminally Ill.* New York: Calvary Hospital.

Salmon, D. (1993) 'Music and emotion in palliative care.' *Journal of Palliative Care 9*, 4, 48–52.

Saunders, C. (1965) 'Watch with me.' *Reprint, Nursing Times,* Nov 26,1.

Saunders, C. (1983) 'The last stages of life.' In C. Corr and D. Corr (eds) *Hospice Care: Principles and Practice.* New York: Springer.

Scher, P. (1996) *Patient-Focused Architecture for Health Care.* Manchester: The Faculty of Art and Design, The Manchester Metropolitan University.

Schloss, G. and Grundy, D. (1994) 'Action techniques in psychopoetry.' In A. Lerner (ed) *Poetry in the Therapeutic Experience.* Saint Louis: MMB Music.

Schnürer, C., Aldridge, D., Altmeier, M., Neugebauer, L., Kleinrath, U. and Steinke, U. (1995) 'Kreativität, Individualität-Wege in der AIDS-Therapie?' *AIDS-FORSCHUNG (AIFO) 10*, 1, 15–35.

Schroeder Sheker, T. (1993) 'Music for the dying: a personal account of the new field of music thanatology: history, theories, and clinical narratives.' *Advances 9*, 1, 36–48.

Seravelli, E. (1988) 'The dying patient, the physician and fear of death.' *New England Journal of Medicine 319*, 26, 1728–1730.

Shapiro, D., Rodrigue, J., Boggs, S. and Robinson, M. (1994) 'Cluster analysis of the Medical Coping Modes Questionnaire – evidence for coping with cancer styles.' *Journal of Psychosomatic Research 38*, 2, 151–159.

Short, A. (1984) *Music Therapy in Hospice Care.* Australian Music Therapy Association Conference Proceedings, Melbourne: Australian Music Therapy Association.

Shoulson, I. (1990) 'Huntington's Disease: Cognitive and psychiatric features.' *Neuropsychiatry, Neuropsychology, and Behavioural Neurology 3*, 15–22.

Sjåsaet, A. (1988) 'Et øyeblikk av frihet.' ('A moment of freedom.') *Musikkterapi 23*, 1, 11–42.

Slivka, H. and Magill, L. (1986) 'The conjoint use of social work and music therapy in working with children of cancer patients.' *Music Therapy 6a*, 1, 30–40.

Sontag, S. (1993). *Krankheit als Metapher.* New York: Fischer.

Sourkes, B. (1982) *The Deepening Shade: Psychological Aspects of Life-Threatening Illness.* Pittsburgh: University of Pittsburgh Press.

Spence, C. (1996) *On Watch – Views from the Lighthouse.* London: Cassell.

Spiegel, D. (1991) 'A psychosocial intervention and survival time of patients with metastatic breast cancer.' *Advances, The Journal of Mind-Body Health 7*, 3, 10–19.

Standley, J. and Hanser, S. (1995) 'Music therapy research and applications in pediatric oncology treatment.' *Journal of Paediatric Oncology Nursing 12*, 1, 3–8, 9–10.

Stanton, A. and Snider, P. (1993) 'Coping with a breast cancer diagnosis: a prospective study.' *Health Psychology 12*, 1, 16–23.

Stedeford, A. (1981) 'Couples facing death.' *British Medical Journal 283*, 1033–1036.

Stige, B. (1993) 'Changes in the music therapy "Space" – with cultural engagement in the local community as an example.' *Nordic Journal of Music Therapy 2*, 2, 11–22.

Storr, A. (1992) *Music and the Mind.* New York: The Free Press.

Strauss, A. and Corbin, J. (1990) *Basics of Qualitative Research: Grounded Theory Procedures and Techniques.* Newbury Park, CA: Sage.

Stubbs, M. (1980) *Language and Literacy: The Sociolinguistics of Reading and Writing*. London: Routledge and Kegan Paul.

Szasz, T. (1998) 'The healing word: its past, present and future.' *Journal of Humanistic Psychology 38*, 2, 8–20.

Tauber, A. (1994) 'A typology of Nietzsche's biology.' *Biology and Philosophy 9*, 25–44.

Tomatis, A. (1996) *The Ear and Language*. Ontario: Moulin Publishing.

Tomm, K. (1990) 'Foreword.' In M. White and D. Epston (eds) *Narrative Means to Therapeutic Ends*. New York: W. W. Norton and Co.

Tsouypoulos, N. (1994) 'Postmodernist theory and the physician-patient relationship.' *Theoretical Medicine 15*, 267–275.

Von Plessen, C. (1995) Krankheitserfahrungen von krebskranken kindern und ihren familien. Unpublished doctoral thesis. Universität Witten/Herdecke.

Walton, J. (1977) *Brain's diseases of the Nervous System*. Oxford: Oxford University Press.

Wear, D. (1993) '"Your breasts/sliced off": literary images of breast cancer.' *Woman and Health 20*, 4, 81–100.

Wenglert, L. and Rosn, A-S. (1995) 'Optimism, self-esteem, mood and subjective health.' *Personal and Individual Difference 18*, 5, 653–661.

White, M. and Epston, D. (1990) *Narrative Means to Therapeutic Ends*. New York: W. W. Norton and Co.

Whitman, W. (1912) *Leaves of Grass and Democratic Vistas*. London: JM Dent and Sons.

Whittall, J. (1989) 'The impact of music therapy in palliative care.' In J. Martin (ed) *The Next Step Forward: Music Therapy with the Terminally Ill*. New York: Calvary Hospital.

Whittall, J. (1991) 'Songs in palliative care: a spouse's last gift.' In K. Bruscia (ed) *Case Studies in Music Therapy*. Phoenixville, PA: Barcelona.

Wilkinson, S. and Kitzinger, C. (1993) 'Whose breast is it anyway? A feminist consideration of advice and "treatment" for breast cancer.' *Women's Studies International Forum 16*, 3, 229–238.

Woodruff, R. (1993) *Palliative Medicine*. Melbourne: Asperula Pty Ltd.

Woodward, J. (1991) *Embracing the Chaos – Theological Responses to AIDS*. London: Society for the Promotion of Christian Knowledge.

Wong, C.A. and Bramwell, L. (1992) 'Uncertainty and anxiety after mastectomy for breast cancer.' *Cancer Nursing 15*, 5, 363–371.

Wylie, M. and Blom, R. (1986) 'Guided imagery and music with hospice patients.' *Music Therapy Perspectives 3*, 25–28.

Zuckerkandl, V. (1973) *Man the Musician – Sound and Symbol: Volume Two*. Princeton, NJ: Princeton University Press.

The Contributors

Trygve Aasgaard is Assistant Professor at Oslo College and a Music Therapist at the Paediatric Department of Ullevål Hospital, The National Hospital and at Lovisenberg Hospice, Norway.

Clare O'Callaghan is a Music Therapist in Victoria, Australia.

Beth Dun is Senior Music Therapist at the Royal Children's Hospital in Melbourne, Australia.

Bridgit Hogan is Chief Music Therapist at Bethlehem Hospital in Victoria, Australia.

Wendy Magee is a Music Therapist at the Royal Hospital for Neuro-disabilty in London.

Susan Weber is Lecturer in Music Therapy at Ludwigs Maximilian University; Music Therapist at the Johannes Hospiz d. Barmherzigen Brüder; Psychologist and Music Therapist at Klinikin Grosshadern in Munich, Germany.

Nigel Hartley is Senior Music Therapist at Sir Michael Sobell House, John Radcliffe NHS Trust, London Lighthouse and the Nordoff-Robbins Centre in London.

Lutz Neugebauer is Music Therapist and Lecturer at the Institute for Music Therapy at the University of Witten/Herdecke, Germany.

Gudrun Aldridge is Music Therapist and Lecturer at the University of Witten/Herdecke, Germany.

Rob Finlayson is a Writer and Researcher in Fremantle, Australia.

Subject Index

Author Index

CPI Antony Rowe
Eastbourne, UK
April 04, 2025